Food Wisdom
for Women

Donna P Feldman MS RDN

The views and information expressed in this book are the views of the author and are not intended to diagnose any medical conditions or to prescribe any treatments. This book is not a replacement for medical advice. The author disclaims responsibility for any loss, liability or risk incurred by use or application of this information.

DEDICATION

To all my friends, family, acquaintances and to the women I don't
know personally, but see everywhere, going about their daily lives, at
the grocery store, at the library, at airports and restaurants and the
rec center and the golf course and walking down the street.
We are all in this big healthy aging experiment together!
This book is for you.
Wishing all of you the best health possible.

CONTENTS

ACKNOWLEDGEMENTS

I have to thank the women who took the time to fill out the questionnaire I used to find out what topics to cover in this book. Frequently health professionals have clear ideas about the topics people *should* want to learn about, but those might not be the topics people *actually* want to learn about. Their input was critical to how I envisioned this book.

1 INTRODUCTION

"Write what you know."

This quote is attributed to Mark Twain, and typically refers to fiction writing. But recently it occurred to me that it's the perfect description of what I wanted to do with this book: write two things I know very well:

- Nutrition
- Being a woman of a certain age. An older age

I definitely know a lot about both of those, both personally and professionally. And strangely there are few books that combine those two areas of expertise in a way that I'd think was useful for the average older woman.

These days nutrition books and blogs are all about pregnancy and organic babies and raising perfectly healthy children, or finding the perfect fad weight loss diet. No one seems to be paying attention to our *very* large, *very* engaged, *very* active and health-conscious generation of older women. Consider this statistic: by the year 2020 it's estimated that there will be more people on the planet over age 65 than under 5. That's remarkable. In the US there will be 80 million people over age 65 by 2040. We've gained about 30 years of life expectancy in the last century. Yet the mass media focus remains on organic babies and yoga moms. Older people are bombarded with ads for prescription drugs.

There's plenty of research on drugs and medical treatments for the common diseases of aging. There isn't much good research on the unique nutritional needs of older people, women in particular. Don't get me wrong: medical treatment can be a marvel and provide plenty of benefits. But medical treatments and medications aren't the basis of fundamental good health. Nutrition is.

Many of the nutrient recommendations for older adults are pure speculation, based on data from studies done decades ago, or from studies on college-aged subjects (always easy to recruit if you're a university-based researcher). When it comes to making recommendations, there's a lot of "Oh we think this is *probably* good enough for people older than 60" kind of thinking. The current controversy about optimal protein intake is one example. There's emerging evidence that older people should consume higher levels than young people, but the powers that be resist changing the official recommended intake.

To some extent, I understand the problems with doing research on older subjects. Older people who volunteer for studies may be a select group, not the average person. People with lots of travel and vacation plans might exclude themselves from long-term studies. People who don't live near research universities won't be included. Older people with existing disease or disabilities, or on certain medications might be excluded by the research design.

Plus there's the issue of study length. For example, a study that truly gave useful information about the benefits of higher protein intake for older people would need to last months, or even years. Everyone would need to be on a controlled measurable diet and controlled exercise plan. If subjects become ill during that time, they might be dropped. If subjects did not adhere to the exercise or diet protocols, they would be dropped. So purely from a logistics point of view, meaningful nutrition studies on older subjects are very problematic.

Which doesn't mean there isn't any useful information out there. Just that it may not be as well supported by research as some people would prefer. It leaves the door open for critics to object to any new ideas. The protein intake controversy is again a good example. Critics can argue the research isn't definitive. It may not be, and that may be because of the limits of recruiting enough people and running a study for a long enough time period.

When I first thought of this book, I had a list of topics in mind based on my professional knowledge of nutrition, as well as on my own personal concerns. But I also wanted input from non-nutrition people – what is important to them? I'm blessed with a group of friends who are also my target audience, so I asked for their thoughts. I know what I think, but maybe they had different concerns.

I wasn't completely surprised to learn that these women were much less interested in disease prevention than in maintaining energy and vitality. Here's how one woman – a novelist -- eloquently put it:

I realized very recently that my goals are to be as healthy as possible and to have what I define as quality of life. For me that is being able to exercise--a lot -- to travel, to enjoy my social groups, write one more novel. My goal is not to prevent heart disease or cancer or diabetes. Doctors work in treatment centers. They treat medical symptoms. What they do not do is give health care. By extension too many articles in AARP promote exercise or supplements or broccoli as "cures." As ways of avoiding death and illness--and life.

So, I would love advice about how to be healthy for its own sake. Because I want to enjoy life and feel as good as possible with an aging body. I want to accept that things are going to break or fail in that body. I might have 70 years or 92, but my goal is to make those years good, not to stretch 70 years to 92.

What I would love is advice that is not fear-based; advice that helps me shape and control my individual health. I would love a book that doesn't promote anything except knowledge. No vegan tirades. No fads. No diets. No condemning dessert, steak or eggs.

And that's precisely what I intend. A book to help you – and me -- to be healthy for health's sake. So that whatever challenges or joys the years throw our way, we can meet them with as much health and energy and vitality as possible.

2 IT'S NOT ALL ABOUT NUTRITION

Before I start writing from the food/nutrition viewpoint, I need to make one thing abundantly clear: your health is *not* all about nutrition.

It's really tempting to think there's a food or supplement solution to all our ills. For some chronic diseases – cardiovascular, hypertension, Type 2 diabetes – diet does indeed play a key role in management. The key word being "diet". There are no magical food or nutrient fixes for these conditions. For other ailments, diet solutions simply don't exist. There are no special diets for tinnitus or Lyme Disease or lower back pain. Despite the claims, there is no known dietary fix for Alzheimer's Disease. Some cancers have a diet connection; many do not. There is no official evidence-based immunity diet, although there are plenty of theories.

I sometimes use the car analogy when talking about nutrition. Your car has many different parts, put together according to a very specific design, and they all have to work together to make the car move. Likewise our bodies have many specific parts and metabolic systems that have to work together to keep us alive and functional. Dumping extra oil over the car engine doesn't make the car run better or faster. Why do we think dumping excessive amounts of vitamins or protein into our bodies makes us healthier?

There are plenty of other factors that impact our health and well being. Some are under our control; some seemingly are not:

- Genetics
- Environment: where we grew up, where we live now
- Social ties
- Cultural norms
- Physical activity
- Random lifestyle factors: where you work, who you live and work with, what you do for leisure time
- Psychological and emotional state

Your genetic background is important, but maybe not as inevitable as you think. The emerging field of epigenetics illustrates how complicated genes can be. You know about DNA, our supposedly hard-wired genetic blueprint. But in fact, DNA is a lot like the keys of a piano. There are 88 keys hardwired into the piano. But do they all play all the time? No. They are played according to written music. Likewise our DNA is "played" according to an extremely complicated set of commands and controls from cells, hormones and tissues. You might have a gene in your DNA for X-effect, but if that gene is never turned on, so what?

Not to get too technical, but it turns out nutrition can play a role the command and control signals that turn genes on or off. At the moment, this is not well understood, but in the future I expect science will reveal many possibilities for influencing gene expression with nutrition. Let's leave it at this: gene expression is a very complicated issue; nutrients certainly have some impact. Someday we'll know more.

Environment is another of those influences that people tend to see as universally negative. Certainly living in a place with horrible air pollution (currently China, for example) or polluted water is a bad thing. Unfortunately people in the developed world seem to have a bleak view of the environment in general. We assume the effects are always unhealthy. We forget about the improvements to air and water quality over the past few decades, not to mention food safety and food abundance.

Social ties and cultural norms are sneaky influencers on health that many people don't recognize. Here's an example: obesity is the new normal. In many parts of the US, and other industrialized countries, obesity is so widespread that people don't even see it anymore. It's just how people look. This has not gone unnoticed by the advertising industry. When a company wants to sell products or services to the Average Person, they tend to use obese actors. Lawn care products, franchise restaurants, pick up trucks, department stores, baby products, household cleaners and on and on – if you use portly actors, the average portly person can relate.

This social/cultural influence has a serious impact on health behaviors. If 90% of the people in your community are overweight/obese, why would you bother to try to lose weight? What support system would you have? Your work environment is part of this, too. If everyone at work is sedentary, there's a box of doughnuts in the break room every morning, people keep bowls of candy on their desks and lunch hour is spent at a local fast food restaurant, how would a lone individual resist that kind of peer pressure every day?

Does stress or anxiety cause you to have stomach pains or headaches or breathing problems? Our emotional and psychological state has an undeniable but poorly understood impact on our health, regardless of nutritional status. Constant stress probably contributes to plenty of health issues, although it's likely wrong to assume stress is the only causative factor. But we all know of people who had a sudden heart problem after a stressful event, or people whose health declined rapidly following the death of a spouse.

What *can* nutrition do?

A healthy diet can help you cope with many of these external assaults, much as a strongly built house can come through a hurricane with little damage compared to a shoddily built house. You can't prevent the hurricane, but at least you can be prepared for it. Likewise eating well can prepare you to deal with life's hurricanes.

But life is not all hurricanes, as you well know. There are plenty of activities for us to enjoy:

Golf	Tennis	Museums
Bridge	Knitting	Painting
Paddleball	Volunteering	Photography
Book clubs	Reading	Singing
Yoga	Dance	Gardening
Horseback riding	Exercise classes	Sewing
Working out	Walking	Dining out
Hiking	Biking	Parties
Discussion groups	Skiing	Concerts
Listening to music	Snowshoeing	Travel
Lunch with friends	Surfing	Playing music
Happy hour with friends	Word games	Book writing
Sudoku	Mah Jong	Swimming
Senior center activities	Needlepoint	Boating
Weaving	Quilting	Fishing
Woodworking	Grandchildren	Movies
Children	Cooking	Picnics
Enrichment classes	College classes	Sports events
Religious activities	Pottery	Pets
A renewed first career	A second career	Shopping

What did I leave out? Highlight the activities you enjoy.

Good nutrition can give you the energy, stamina, and vitality to keep on enjoying all those things that make your life worth living, things that get you up in the morning, things that make you smile.

Nutrition Status

Here's something that frustrates me. There's no test for "nutrition status". So how can you tell your body is in good nutritional shape? At the moment, you can't.

Certainly you can't tell just be looking at a person that they're consuming optimal amounts of all known nutrients. For one thing, scientists can't agree on what "optimal" means. Intake recommendations are based on amounts that should be adequate for the vast majority of people. Many of these numbers are based on results from small scale studies done many years ago, typically on young men (women have that problematic menstrual cycle that could complicate results). And some of those studies were designed to create extreme deficiencies of just one vitamin in a short period of time, a situation that rare, if ever, occurs in real life. So while it's interesting to find that having almost no B1 intake leads to certain dramatic symptoms, how does that help the average person?

Then there's the problem of intake vs. blood or tissue levels. Before a nutrient can provide any benefit, it has to be absorbed. If someone is malabsorbing some nutrient, their intake might look adequate, but in fact their status will not be. Vitamin B12 is a great example of this problem. Absorption of this vitamin is controlled by a specific molecule, intrinsic factor. Some people lack this key molecule due to genetic or other issues. They might have a great intake of B12, but in fact their actual B12 status is poor. And they might not know until problems develop that are linked to B12 deficiency. At which point a physician might order a blood test for B21 status. Or might not, attributing the symptoms to something else, because it sounds like you're eating a sufficient amount of B12-rich foods. Oops. Key Message: intake alone might not always be meaningful.

You might think: just have a blood test for all known nutrients. For some nutrients, that might work, but it would be expensive. And blood tests might not be the best test for all nutrients. Calcium is a good example of that problem. Blood calcium has to be maintained within a narrow range *No Matter*

What. Calcium is a key player in many metabolic functions, such as muscle contraction and blood clotting. Blood levels can't be allowed to fluctuate based on intake from day to day. So blood calcium is controlled by a system of hormones. If inadequate calcium is absorbed from your diet, the hormones send messages to your bones to release calcium. You can't look at your blood test results for calcium and conclude "Oh, I'm consuming enough calcium, because it's normal."

Then there's the question of "optimal". I can't think of any nutrient for which there is an official *optimal* intake. The word optimal implies some level of perfection that no one wants to commit to publicly, because we don't know how to define it. Instead we have "adequate", enough of a nutrient to meet some basic level of needs for basic health. Above which there isn't much more benefit. Below which you start to have problems.

Vitamin D is a good example of this problem. Over the past several years, vitamin D has grabbed the attention of researchers, doctors and the general public. People are taking supplements; researchers are investigating D for miracle cure properties, with unconvincing results. There's some agreement about what constitutes a deficient blood level; there's much less about what "adequate" or "optimal" are. In fact, different medical laboratories can have different normal ranges for vitamin D.

One more thing

I need to clarify one more thing that nutrition alone cannot do: it can't create fitness. I'll have more on muscles and energy later in the book, but suffice it to say just eating well, particularly boosting protein intake, does not build muscles or improve fitness. You need to move those muscles and you need to be consistent about it. You also need to choose the right levels of activity, not overdoing exercises, but pushing yourself in an appropriate manner for your age, starting fitness level, your goals and health status. If you're unsure what to do or where to start, try to find a qualified trainer or perhaps a physical therapist who can help you set up a plan. If your town or city has a recreational center or senior center, you will likely find resources there to help you get going.

Don't worry about wearing stylish workout clothes or looking like the actors in TV ads for sports drinks. Exercise isn't just for muscular 20-somethings, sweating out some high speed spin class, or lifting hundreds of pounds of weights while wearing cute headbands and tight pants. Normal people working out at gyms and rec centers are more concerned about doing their own workout than looking like a TV actor. The people –old and young -- who work out and take classes at my rec center come in a variety of body types, wearing comfortable clothes, all doing their own thing to stay fit.

Finally, there is no "perfect" activity that you must do. If you prefer gentle yoga, don't feel guilty about not using weight machines. If you prefer the stationary bike because you can read while biking, don't feel guilty about not riding outside. You should enjoy your activities, or at least feel good about completing them. I don't particularly look forward to my workout with weight machines, but I know I need to use them on a regular basis to maintain strength and muscle tone. I always feel better about it on the way home. The best description might be "empowered". If you can feel empowered after completing a workout, that's something positive.

3 MENOPAUSE

We're all in this together

If you're reading this book, it's likely you're either done with the menopause transition or are going through it. For all the women who have moved beyond that period, I have one question: would you want to go back to having periods every month? Dealing with hormonal changes? Mood swings? Monthly weight swings? As you move past menopause, all of that starts to seem like another world.

According to a study done more than 2 years ago, some one *billion* women around the globe have gone through menopause. While all these women experience this transition differently, according to their social and cultural expectations, the most common physical symptoms are hot flashes and night sweats.

Unlike diabetes or cancer, menopause is not a medical condition. It's a natural and inevitable part of aging. But it is accompanied by physical symptoms that can range from annoying to disruptive. For some women, quality of life can deteriorate, if only temporarily. Other women cope with minor but annoying symptoms until they resolve, and then move on with life.

The major driver of menopause is loss of hormones. The most significant outcome of this change is that menstrual periods cease. But the decreasing hormones contribute to physical symptoms, such as hot flashes and night sweats, which can lead to sleep disruption and fatigue. Bone loss is another possible outcome, although it's not obvious except with a bone scan. There's a general expectation that menopause causes weight gain. But weight gain can also be a side effect of sleep disruption and fatigue, which can impact metabolism, exercise and food choices.

What does research say? There's compelling evidence that symptoms like hot flashes are worse for women who are obese or are smokers. A possible explanation: as estrogen levels fall, fat cells are more prone to releasing pro-inflammatory molecules. So if you are obese you have more fat cells releasing those inflammatory mediators, worsening symptoms like hot flashes.

Other studies find that women with the worst symptoms have the highest risk for developing Type 2 diabetes or heart disease. But of course, excess weight is a major risk factor for those chronic diseases. So what's more likely is that excess body fat puts older women at risk for:

1. More severe menopause symptoms
2. Development of chronic diseases associated with age

The topic of menopause and diet/nutrition can be divided into two parts:

Phase 1: going through the menopause transition, as hormone levels fall causing unpleasant and bothersome physical symptoms.

Phase 2: the rest of your life, after the transition is over, your menstrual periods have ceased, your hormones have leveled off and symptoms subside.

Phase 1 gets most of the diet/nutrition attention, as people look for ways to alleviate symptoms. Phase 2 gets less special attention. Hot flashes, night sweats and other noticeable discomforts have dissipated. But in fact, this is a critical time to focus on the best diet and nutrition possible. After menopause, you're more at risk for heart disease, hypertension, muscle loss and frailty, cognitive decline, bone loss and other problems associated with aging. Nutrition impacts all of these concerns. You might not notice muscle loss or thinning bones the way you notice night sweats and a headache. That doesn't mean you can just wait for serious problems to develop before taking action.

This book is mostly about the nutrition and food strategies you can implement for Phase 2, to enhance your quality of life and your health. But before you get to that phase, you have to go through the menopause transition. What are some of the nutrition strategies for that time of life?

Phase 1

There are plenty of food, herb, nutrition and diet recommendations for alleviation of menopause symptoms. Some women swear by them; others experienced no benefit. Of course, we hear about the positive anecdotes, especially if they're used to sell a product. Miracle cures for menopause symptoms include:

- foods like flax seed, soy and yams (or sweet potatoes)
- herbs like black cohosh, St. John's Wort, ginseng, sage and red clover
- nutrients like vitamin D, vitamin E, omega-3

So far, the evidence for actual benefit (reduced symptoms) is intriguing (soy), minimal (flax) or absent (yam). Some of the recommended herbs can have adverse side effects. Black cohosh can cause liver toxicity. Never take any herbal menopause supplements without first discussing with your physician, or, if you are on long term medications, with a pharmacist.

Soy is a rich source of isoflavones, which are phytoestrogens – plant-sourced estrogen-like compounds. So when it comes to dealing with menopause symptoms caused by falling hormone levels, soy foods have gotten lots of attention. The isoflavones genistein and daidzein have mild estrogen-like activity.

One recent study compared 40 mg daily doses of soy isoflavones to conventional hormone replacement therapy

(HRT) for relief of symptoms. After 1 year, women taking either HRT or isoflavones reported significantly reduced symptom severity compared to a control group. Other studies find that isoflavones may be only half as potent as HRT and take more time to become effective.

When it comes to symptom relief, studies suggest genistein seems to be the more potent isoflavone. However, an isoflavone metabolite, equol, can also alleviate menopausal symptoms. There's a catch. Equol is not found in food; it's produced when gut microbes metabolize daidzein. Only about 25-30% of women in Western countries are so-called "equol producers," meaning when they consume daidzein from soy foods, it is metabolized to equol. Interestingly, that percentage of equol producers is doubled for vegetarians and for women in Asian countries. The reason for this isn't clear; is it particular gut microbes or genetics or overall diet or some interaction of all three? It does explain why some women who deliberately add more soy foods to their diets will get more relief from menopausal symptoms than others who eat the same soy foods. Meanwhile researchers can bypass this source of confusion by using equol supplements in studies.

In fact, most of these studies use soy isoflavones supplements rather than soy foods like tofu, edamame or soy milk. This isn't surprising; supplements with measured doses make for better data. But high daily intake of these phytoestrogens typically depends on food. Average intake of isoflavones ranges from 25-50 mg/day in Asian countries like Japan, with some people regularly consuming up to 100 mg/day. In Western countries, intake averages a mere 1-2 mg/day.

Should you eat more soy? This question isn't answered without some controversy. Years ago, soy was on the health food radar screen because it supposedly helped prevent breast cancer. Not long after that, it was blamed for breast cancer. Where does this controversy stand today? In short we don't have definitive answers.

One problem with studying the impact of soy on any health condition is the wide range of possible soy foods and varying content of soy isoflavones in those foods. As noted above, the isoflavone genistein can have different effects than diadzein, which may be metabolized to equol. Cells growing in labs that are treated with isoflavones may behave quite differently than cells in the body, making it hard to extrapolate lab findings to the real world.

Add to that the fact that we have greatly expended understanding of the different types of breast cancer cells, which respond differently to hormone signals. Certain soy isoflavones may be helpful for one women, but not for another, based on cancer type. No wonder women may be hesitant to add soy to their diets to lessen annoying menopause symptoms.

There's one additional clue from population studies: women in Asian countries who grow up eating lots of soy foods throughout life have a significantly lower rate of breast cancer compared to women in Western countries. Is it just the soy, or is it the whole diet? Or genetics? One thing we could conclude is that, if soy did increase risk for breast cancer, rates in Asian countries would be very high.

The key point is that in Asian countries, soy is consumed as soy foods, not as capsules of isolated soy extracts. If you were considering soy as an intervention for menopause symptoms, increasing soy foods is a preferable strategy. Until we know more about the metabolic activity of the different soy isoflavones, as well as more about the impact of gut bacteria, eating more soy foods may be the best approach. The soy foods with the highest isoflavone content are:

- Soy flour
- Soy protein
- Soy beans
- Tofu
- Tempeh
- Miso
- Soy milk and soy cheeses

Some non-soy foods like split peas and peanuts also have some isoflavone content, although not nearly as much as soy.

Other Strategies

Other than increasing soy, what else can you do? When it comes to hot flashes, night sweats and other vasomotor symptoms caused by menopause, some women find relief by avoiding certain foods and beverages. Some common culprits include:

- Wine, especially red wine
- Other alcoholic beverages
- Hot spicy foods
- Caffeine
- Other stimulants found in some herb teas or foods like chocolate.
- Cured meats
- MSG
- Tomato, especially cooked tomato products

These are the obvious culprits. It's entirely possible that none of these bother you. Or you may notice that other foods worsen your symptoms, or that symptoms are only worsened when you consume several of these together at one meal.

Alcohol in general may be especially problematic for older women, as our ability to metabolize alcohol decreases with age. You might notice you just can't drink an amount you used to tolerate 30 years ago. That's normal.

Because nutrients like vitamin D and omega-3 are important for general health, they could help by improving the overall health status of women who were deficient. But no single nutrients have been identified (thus far) that clearly decrease menopause symptoms.

Until medical science comes up with additional information, the best strategy within your control is:

- Keep weight in normal range
- Stay active
- Avoid foods you believe aggravate symptoms
- Add soy foods if you desire
- Eat a well balanced, plant-based diet that includes

probiotic foods and maximizes nutrient intake.
- Stay hydrated.

Phase 2

Once you get beyond the menopause transition, your symptoms should subside. Benefits: you don't get menstrual periods anymore! But now you need to pay special attention to diet and exercise as your first line of defense against the increasing risk older women have for heart disease, osteoporosis, Type 2 diabetes, hypertension and cancer.

But it's not all about simply fending off diseases. Diet and nutrition impact many quality-of-life issues for older women, everything from eye health to brain function to digestion, strength, energy and weight management. The rest of this book addresses many of those issues, arming you with information you can use to make this whole aging process more of an adventure. We older women are a vanguard, leading the charge to turn the conventional view of aging on its proverbial head. Arm yourself with health!

4 HYDRATION

My house is not air conditioned. We live in a climate that can get extremely hot on summer days, with a dry unrelenting heat, but then the temperatures cool off at night. For years, I just coped with it without issue. But then something changed. While sitting at the computer I noticed a slightly woozy feeling, like the heat was just *getting* to me. Not pleasant at all and rather strange, because I drink plenty of fluids. I assumed my usual fluid intake was sufficient.

I mentioned my discomfort to a friend of the same age, who lives nearby and she reported feeling the same way. And she had air conditioning! Something was 'off' because of the extreme heat. But what?

When heat waves strike, especially in major cities, we always hear about heat-related deaths, especially among the elderly. Now I don't feel particularly 'elderly', but I accept that at this stage of my life, some of those elderly-type physical changes are happening. One of those is trouble maintaining proper hydration.

Hydration and Aging

There is an emerging body of knowledge about hydration in older people. There's good evidence that fluid balance starts to go 'off' a bit as we age. Normally your body is 50-65% water, depending on how much fat tissue (lower water content) you have. Every metabolic system, from digestion to muscle movement to breathing to energy metabolism to thinking happens in a water-based medium. We all need the proper fluid balance in order to function. It's one of the most basic needs.

Ideally water intake and output balance out on a daily basis. Input isn't just water you drink. Water intake comes from all beverages, from milk to juice to soft drinks, from high water content vegetables and fruits, from cooked grains or pasta and even some from meats. Water output is in urine and feces, sweat, water vapor in your breath and some constant low level loss from your skin. On average you might turn over 3-4 quarts of water a day. An athlete might need 10 quarts sweating in a warm environment.

What's that water doing in your body? Water is inside all your cells, outside your cells in extracellular fluid compartments, and in your blood, which is 80% water. The amount of fluid in all these places is regulated by hormones and feedback mechanisms that sense blood pressure or blood concentration and send messages to the kidneys to alter water or sodium loss and to the brain to signal thirst when necessary.

Why is this a problem?

So what happens when age and hot weather intersect? The theory is that, with age, our thirst response becomes less sensitive and kidney function is less responsive to the hormone signals calling for water conservation. In hot weather, we sweat to cool off. The sweat might evaporate quickly, so you don't have the sensation of sweat running down your face or back, which might be a signal to drink more water. You might also lose more water vapor from breathing as well as more non-sweat loss through skin. If fluid loss is not replaced, we gradually become dehydrated, yet the signals to conserve water (kidneys) and drink more water (brain) aren't working so well. Result: gradual fluid depletion and dehydration.

For older people, medications may complicate this picture further. And water itself might be an issue if you don't like the taste of your water or don't always have access to water. Or are forgetful and so don't drink more water consistently.

Recent studies on nursing home residents measured hydration status using serum osmolality, a measure of blood concentration. The more concentrated your blood, the more dehydrated you are. One study found that over 1/3 of the nursing home residents were dehydrated and an additional 30% had impending dehydration.

Dehydration that raises serum osmolality causes water to be moved from inside cells into blood, to correct the high concentration. Now your cells are dehydrated, with less fluid than is ideal for metabolic functions. Feedback mechanisms should trigger thirst, but with age, our thirst response is impaired. Kidneys are less able to conserve water. Dehydration continues.

What happens then? Especially in hot weather, you have less body water available for sweating, so you are less able to regulate body temperature. You might become overheated even if you aren't physically active. Blood pressure may be adversely impacted. Dehydration impacts everything, from cognitive function to energy level and fine motor skills. In short, you don't feel well.

What To Do

If you've noticed that hot weather is getting to you more than in the past, you might be experiencing the effects of aging on fluid balance. The first best plan is to avoid dehydration in the first place, all year long. You don't need to drink dramatically huge amounts of water. The adage about 8 glasses a day is a nice general purpose recommendation, if only to act as a reminder of the importance of fluid intake. Some people may be comfortable with more or less than that. You may need to bump that up during very hot weather. Certain medications may affect fluid balance; your nurse or physician should discuss that with you.

Here are some ideas to ensure adequate water intake:

1. Create visual or physical cues to drink more water. Get a water bottle or pitcher or other container that sits in view so you remember to drink.
2. If you don't like plain water, find other beverages. Herbal tea and black tea can be iced or hot. Coffee is another option. The idea that coffee is dehydrating has been dispelled by research, although that information hasn't always trickled down to the consumer level. Seltzer water or club soda are also options.
3. Don't rely on alcoholic beverages for hydration! Alcohol *is* dehydrating. If you drink alcohol anytime, drink plain water or other nonalcoholic beverage along with it even when weather isn't hot.
4. Include plenty of high water content vegetables and fruits in your diet especially during hot weather. Luckily many of these are fresh and in season during those times of year. Think cucumbers, melons, peppers, peaches, plums, berries, lettuces and tomatoes.
5. Have one or more water bottles ready for times you're out and about: for your car, your purse, your golf bag, your knitting bag.

What about salt?

A discussion of hydration isn't really complete without some mention of salt. Most of us are aware that salt intake has some impact on fluid balance. People frequently complain that they're retaining fluid because they ate salty food. Your kidneys will flush out excess sodium (from salt), but only if you drink enough water to make that happen.

Salt intake is one of the most controversial nutrition topics of the 21st Century. Why do we care about salt? Because it is the major source of sodium in our diets. High sodium intake is associated with hypertension. Major public health organizations, such as the American Heart Association, advocate very, very low sodium intake, assuming this will fix hypertension.

The current recommended limit – 1500 mg of sodium/day – would pretty much exclude foods like bread and cheese, not to mention salad dressings, fast food, cured meats and soy sauce. But other scientists and organization are pushing back on extreme this salt limit, suggesting that a moderate recommendation of 2500 mg, or even 3000, is fine for the vast majority of people. I don't expect this controversy to go away anytime soon.

I write about sodium and salt on a regular basis in my blog, Radio Nutrition. My professional point of view is this: the focus on salt does nothing to address other nutritional issues that can impact health and risk for high blood pressure. Potassium intake is a critical piece of the blood pressure puzzle, but that's never addressed. Potassium and sodium must be in balance. Potassium comes primarily from vegetables, fruits and whole grains, foods lacking in the typical high sodium diet. So is it the sodium, or the lack of potassium?

Sodium and potassium work together in our bodies to balance fluids inside and outside cells. There is a type of dehydration caused by loss of sodium from the body, usually from a disease process like vomiting or diarrhea. Heavy and prolonged sweating can also result in sodium loss. People working in underground mines, wild land firefighters and endurance athletes are examples of people who may lose too much sodium in sweat.

In these extreme situations, simply drinking more water without also replacing sodium and potassium can be dangerous. You might not be a wild land fire fighter, but you could lose excess sodium during a severe bout of vomiting/diarrhea caused by an infection such as norovirus or listeria. In these situations, a sports drink or some soup can help you get back to normal. Your physician may have other recommendations. But unless you are competing in a marathon or working outdoors for hours on an extremely hot day or have been losing fluid and electrolytes due to an illness, you probably don't need to be concerned about sodium loss. Dehydration will typically be related to inadequate fluid intake.

My approach to salt

I don't deliberate restrict or obsess about my salt intake. I rarely eat salty commercial foods, like chips or cured meats, salted nuts or fast food. I eat lots of high potassium vegetables and fruits. I shake a dash of salt on foods like potatoes, fresh tomatoes, green salad, meats, eggs and chicken. If I were in an extreme hot weather situation where I was sweating a lot and drinking an unusual amount of water, I might deliberately add a salty food to my diet.

What should you do? Your physician will instruct you to restrict salt as necessary for high blood pressure or kidney disease. Avoiding highly processed foods is a simple strategy for reducing salt intake. I always recommend plenty of high potassium fruits and vegetables anyway, since they contain lots of other nutrients that you won't find in chips or nacho cheese sauce. Some of the best potassium sources are:

- Potatoes
- Legumes (kidney beans, black beans, etc)
- Soy beans
- Tomatoes
- Dried fruit such as apricots, peaches, figs, raisins, currants
- Bananas
- Greens
- Peanuts and other nuts
- Oranges, grapefruit and other citrus
- Juice of citrus fruits
- Yams and sweet potato
- Whole grains
- Milk

Most other vegetables and fruits are decent sources of potassium.

5 STRONG BONES

If there's one age-related health issue women in our age range have had drummed into our consciousness it's *bone health*. The specter of prolonged disability caused by a broken bone is our worst nightmare. So of course we want strong bones. The medical industry has obligingly developed tests to encourage (scare?) us into taking drugs that are supposed to ward off this problem. The supplement industry chimes in with calcium supplements. The dairy industry chimes in with promotion of high calcium dairy foods. Other food manufacturers slap a health halo on beverages like orange juice and soy milk by adding calcium to the mix. We're encouraged to engage in weight bearing exercise, which supposedly stimulates bones to stay strong.

Bones 101

Bones are not just blocks of calcium. They are living tissue, constantly renewing, even after skeletal growth has stopped. Yes calcium is important, but many other nutrients are essential to bone strength, including:

- Protein
- Potassium
- Phosphorus
- Magnesium
- Boron
- Copper
- Zinc
- Vitamin D
- Vitamin K (likely)
- Vitamin B12 (possibly)
- Vitamin C (possibly, needed for synthesis of collagen, which is part of bone matrix)

Simply taking a calcium supplement and calling it a day on bone health is not a great plan. What about all those other nutrients? Even so-called bone supplements do not have all those nutrients. It would be an enormous pill in any event, impossible to swallow.

Bones give structure to our bodies, but they also serve as a reservoir for calcium, which is essential for many other metabolic systems. Muscle contraction depends on calcium. Calcium is involved with enzyme systems and blood clotting. In other words, calcium is essential for life and your blood level is maintained regardless of intake. Having a reservoir for times when calcium intake is poor is your body's back up plan. Hormones signal bones to release more calcium to prop up your blood level. But if the poor intake goes on for too long, bones start to demineralize, leading to osteopenia and osteoporosis, which weakens bones and can lead to fractures and interfere with fracture repair.

The bone matrix

Bone density refers to the degree of mineralization of bones. Think of bones as a complicated matrix, sort of like a bird's nest made of twigs and stems. The nest is made stronger as the birds pack that matrix with mud or other substances that fill in the matrix of twigs and harden.

Your bones are structured like that, in a manner of speaking. The matrix is collagen, made of protein, which gives strength and also flexibility to bones. The matrix is hardened by a filling of mineral salt deposits. One major component is hydroxyapatite, a complex mineral salt made of calcium and phosphorus. Other mineral salts, such as magnesium and potassium, help to stabilize the hydroxyapatite.

Normally, two sets of specialized cells and enzyme systems are at work in bones:

1. Bone Formation: Special cells called osteoblasts control formation of new bone matrix.
2. Bone Resorption, or breakdown: Osteoclasts secrete enzymes that degrade bone matrix and mineral salts, which are then released into blood for use elsewhere.

Bone resorption might sound like a bad thing, but in fact it's important for bone health throughout life. Bones are not inert blocks; they undergo constant repair and renewal. Resorption is critical for this bone remodeling process, which maintains the integrity of bone structure and is a key part of fracture repair. As the bone resorption process removes old tissue, the bone formation system moves in to replace it with new healthy tissue so bones stay strong and resilient.

Bones grow in length and strength from birth. Assuming healthy intake of bone building nutrients, bone mass peaks sometime around age 30. Of course, plenty of factors can interfere, such as:

- Chronic low calcium diet in childhood and adolescence
- Imbalances of hormones that affect bone formation
- The nutritional demands of pregnancy and lactation, especially multiple pregnancies at young age
- Inadequate intake of vitamin D, and poor calcium absorption

Past age 30, we experience gradual loss of bone density that accelerates once we hit menopause. Estrogen helps to keep minerals in bones, and once it drops off, bone density typically goes down. How much density you lose depends on genetics, nutrition and other factors.

DEXA bone scans measure the density of minerals in your bones. They are recommended for women over age 65, and for younger women who have known risk factors for osteoporosis. If the scan indicates your bones have suboptimal mineralization, you may be told to increase calcium intake and perhaps also take a medication that increases bone density. These medications work by interfering with bone resorption, favoring the bone formation system, to push calcium into bones. One result is that the renewal and repair process of bone remodeling is suppressed.

Bone Nutrition Plan

The best plan for bone health in older age would of course be to maintain bone strength throughout life. That way, the inevitable bone loss after menopause will not have a dramatic impact. But many of us arrive at that time of life with bones that have already lost significant mineralization for a variety of commonplace reasons:

- Poor calcium intake, perhaps for years, complicated by the demands of multiple pregnancies and lactation.
- Long-term unrecognized vitamin D insufficiency
- Poor intake of other key bone nutrients, such as magnesium and potassium
- Lack of weight bearing exercise that stimulates bones to stay strong
- Genetic factors also work against many of us. If you know female relatives in older generations had osteoporosis, or experienced debilitating hip or other fractures, you might also have that genetic predisposition.
- Loss of menstrual periods due to anorexia or excessive exercise. When menstruation shuts down, it's a sign that hormones have been impacted by insufficient food intake. Anorexia and over-training can have the same impact on hormones, and sometimes go hand in hand. Bone strength can be severely impacted for the long term, due to poor intake and hormone imbalance, even if the person eventually recovers body weight.

Can you rebuild bone health in later years? Yes, although perhaps not up to the level of a 30 year old, but strong enough to resist fractures more effectively.

The most effective strategy you can adopt on your own is to boost intake of all bone nutrients across the board. This doesn't mean going crazy over any particular nutrient. It does mean paying attention and planning a bone enhancing diet. What would that include?

Vitamin D

First you need to be sure you've got sufficient vitamin D on board because vitamin D controls calcium absorption. Most doctors now do routine vitamin D blood tests as part of a yearly wellness check up. Be sure you get that test, so you know where you stand in terms of vitamin D sufficiency. You can supplement if necessary. Don't just take supplements blindly. See the Vitamin D section in the Chapter 12 for more information on that.

Calcium

In the US, older women are advised to consume 1200 mg of calcium a day. Other Westernized countries have similar recommendations. Asian countries tend to have lower calcium recommendations. US food intake data show that older women average 850 mg calcium a day from food. Women who take supplements (about ¼ of the population) average another 750 mg from those.

It's entirely possible to get sufficient calcium from food. You would likely consume dairy products every day, or use foods fortified with calcium, such as soy milk, and/or eat lots of higher calcium vegetables like greens or legumes. Here's a general list of high calcium foods:

- Milk (cow, sheep, goat)
- Cheese
- Yogurt
- kefir
- Tofu (made with calcium sulfate process)
- Soy milk fortified with calcium
- Legumes (cooked dried beans)
- Orange juice fortified with calcium
- Plant "milks" fortified with calcium
- Greens, such as collards, spinach, turnip, kale, chard

Some unexpected foods have significant calcium, although you might not eat them that frequently: rhubarb, canned sardines (you eat the bones), taro root and canned salmon (again, bones). Calcium might be added to processed foods like breakfast cereals and meal replacement or snack bars.

Some nuts, particularly almonds and sesame seeds, are decent calcium sources. But you would have to eat a lot of calories to get significant calcium. The amount of calcium in 5 TB of tahini or 1-1/4 cup almonds equals the amount in one cup of low fat milk. But that means consuming 450 calories from tahini or 800 from almonds vs. 110 from milk. If you need to gain weight or you're hiking the PCT à la "Wild," and need the calories, nuts might be a preferred calcium source.

Most other foods have at least some calcium, so if you eat 3 or more servings of high calcium foods, your total intake could be in the 1000-1200 mg/day range, which is excellent. But of course the key is that this has to be an everyday effort.

One more catch: the form of calcium in plant foods like greens is less easily absorbed than the calcium in dairy foods. So relying entirely on plant foods might result in less available calcium, depending on your digestive system.

Some people just aren't going to eat so many higher calcium foods every day, in which case a supplement can help you maintain an adequate intake. Supplements typically come in 300 mg doses, which is roughly the equivalent of one serving of a dairy food. I don't recommend just relying on supplements. Food has all kinds of other nutrients lacking in a calcium supplement. If you included 1-2 high calcium foods daily and added one supplement, you could attain an intake of about 1000 mg/day.

Absorption studies show that you can't absorb more than about 500 mg of calcium at any one time, so taking a calcium supplement with a glass of milk or fortified orange juice may be wasteful. Calcium intake should be spread out as evenly as possible throughout the day.

Phosphorus

Everyone worries about calcium, but phosphorus should have equal billing when it comes to bone mineralization. Phosphorus makes up over half the mass of bone minerals, yet no one talks about it. Maybe because there is no one food group that's especially high phosphorus, as there is with calcium (dairy foods), turning the nutrient into a marketing tool. Phosphorus is in almost all food, with the exception of fats, oils and sugar. No marketing benefit to be had.

The importance of phosphorus is a good argument for getting calcium from foods rather than supplements, since foods will also contain phosphorus. Highest sources include meats, nuts, whole grains, legumes and dairy foods.

Protein

Protein has to come from food. Eating more than you need isn't going to help. You can't force bones or muscles to grow by loading up on protein. You probably know that meats, poultry, eggs and dairy foods are high protein foods. Plant protein foods include nuts, legumes, soy foods and, to a lesser extent, whole grains.

Dairy foods are promoted for bone health because of the calcium content, but they're also an excellent source of protein, phosphorus, potassium, and zinc, and are typically fortified with vitamin D. All of these nutrients are important for bone strength, so if you like dairy foods, your bones will benefit.

Soy milk is also a good protein source, but be sure to pick brands fortified with calcium (most are). Soy milk is also a good source of those other bone nutrients.

Other plant milks – almond, coconut, rice, etc. – are *not* high protein. Some are also poor sources of phosphorus and potassium, so while they may be fortified with calcium, soy or animal-sourced milks are better choices if you want to maximize nutrient content.

Everything else

As you can see from the list at the beginning of the chapter, a wide variety of nutrients are critical for bone health: minerals, protein and vitamins. The catch for older women is that, with age, energy needs decrease. You've probably noticed that you eat less than you did at age 30, yet you still need the same nutrient intake. In some cases, such as for calcium you need *more.* Which means your food choices must be increasingly nutrient-dense. There's less room for treats or empty calories.

Unfortunately, for some of us this is also a time when diet could drift towards more ready-to-eat processed foods. Cooking can be a chore; you may be busy with other things. Taste preferences change. Nutrient intake may end up sub-par.

So for the 'everything else' part of bone health, it might make sense to add a multiple vitamin/mineral to your strategy. I've got more information about those in the Supplements chapter. But here's the argument in short: your diet needs to be more nutrient dense. You might be able to achieve that most of the time, but not all of the time. Or some perfectly wholesome foods might not appeal to, or agree with you anymore, limiting intake of some nutrients. A multiple can fill in the gaps. You don't even need to take it everyday, since the point is to *supplement* your intake of nutrients, not replace it.

How do you know it's working?

The only way to know if your nutrient-dense diet has rewarded you with mineral-dense bones is with a DEXA scan. Those typically are done every two years at most, since it takes months for bones to build up. So there really isn't an easy quick way to see if you're making progress.

If you already know your bones are in good shape, just maintaining your diet as-is should be fine, as long as some other medical issue doesn't impact bone health. If you've had a scan that indicated thinning bones, whether osteopenia or osteoporosis, you should plan to boost your intake of calcium and stick to a well balanced diet, with supplements added if appropriate. If you have not had a scan, but suspect you could develop a problem, then improving your diet is a very good idea. Factors to consider include:

- family history
- years of poor intake of calcium and other bone nutrients
- other factors in your health history, such as periods of amenorrhea
- a history of easily broken bones

If you start medication intended to increase bone density, you definitely need to pay attention to calcium intake. As noted above, the medications work by pushing calcium into bones. So you need to consume that calcium; it doesn't appear in your blood magically. In fact, medications instructions should provide information about that.

The main take-away message is that, medication or not, if you have thinning bones, your current diet is not adequate to maintain bone health, and you need to make some changes.

6 STRENGTH

Years ago, you vowed that aging would not slow you down. You would keep up with jogging, biking, walking, swimming, sports and dancing. You haven't gained weight. You look forward to playing with grandchildren. But somehow despite working out and eating well, you slow down. You don't feel like you have the strength or agility you once had. What happened?

Sarcopenia, or the slow inevitable loss of muscle mass with age, may be the culprit. Sarcopenia can contribute to a loss of mobility and strength, upwards of 3% per year after age 60. It can eventually contribute to frailty and increased risk for falls and fractures. Adding insult to injury, you may weigh the same as 20 years ago and think everything is fine. But with sarcopenia, more of your body is fat and less is muscle. And a higher percent of body fat creates other health risks.

As the world population ages, the quality-of-life problems and potential adverse health effects of sarcopenia loom large. At the moment, there isn't even a standard way to diagnose it. Agencies in some countries are working on simple screening tests. But screening doesn't answer the basic question: why does it happen and what can be done about it?

Muscles 101

In order to understand sarcopenia, it's important to understand basic muscle biology. Muscles are made up of fibers, which come in two types:

Fast twitch: contract quickly; tire quickly; used for rapid movement such as sprinting or jumping.

Slow twitch: good for endurance activity; can work longer before fatigue sets in.

Movement of the fast and slow twitch fibers in your muscles is controlled by neurons. These neurons deteriorate as we age, causing the affected muscle fibers to atrophy. When neurons to fast twitch fibers die, other neurons that feed slow twitch fibers can grow to take their place. But now the muscle ends up working less effectively because slow twitch neurons fire more slowly and with less power. Your capacity for fast movements, whether dashing after a grandchild or quickly catching your balance, is impaired. This is one classic aspect of sarcopenia.

Like bones, muscle tissue integrity is maintained by a process of constant repair and replacement throughout life. As we age, the synthesis part of this equation decreases. In other words, muscle breakdown continues, but muscle repair doesn't keep up. Growth hormone, testosterone and other hormones affect muscle regeneration, and those also decline with age, adding to the problem.

Muscle regeneration can't happen in a vacuum. It depends on the quantity and quality of the protein you eat. But eating loads of protein isn't the whole answer either. You have to use your muscles, meaning both the neurons that send the signals and the muscle fibers that do the work. Muscles that are used are stimulated to maintain integrity; muscles that are not used are more likely to lose mass. Muscle loss can be measured after just a few days of inactivity. This is an especially important point for older women, who might experience periods of inactivity due to illness or other circumstances.

Muscle Nutrition

Muscles are made from the protein we eat. Protein in food is broken down into the amino acid building blocks, which are absorbed. They travel to different tissues in your body, and are used to assemble proteins for a multitude of uses, from muscle fiber to enzymes to hormones and signaling molecules to cell structures and hemoglobin, to name a few.

Twenty-two amino acids make up the proteins we eat. Of those 22, nine are considered essential, meaning the human body cannot synthesize any of them. We must consume a certain quantity, on average, every day. For example, for a 150 lb adult woman who needs a minimum of 55 grams of total protein a day, 5-6 grams should be essential amino acids. Because we eat mixed meals, we don't really have to think about this requirement as a separate thing. For example, the protein in milk or egg is about 50% essential amino acids, so those foods contribute significantly to meeting your requirement.

Some people have to pay more attention to protein in foods, mainly vegans. Plant foods have less protein, and that protein tends to have unbalanced ratios of the essential amino acids. Combining plant foods with different ratios of essential amino acids, such as grains and legumes, helps to improve protein quality and quantity. Soy is one exception. Soy has significant protein that's also high quality. Foods made with soy, such as tofu or soy milk, are good protein sources.

How much protein do we need?

The standard recommended protein intake for adults is 0.8 grams protein per kilogram body weight per day. When it comes to older adults, this number is increasingly controversial. Studies on older adults hint that higher protein intakes may be beneficial, especially as a strategy for preventing or combating sarcopenia.

Where did the 0.8 gram number come from? It came from so-called nitrogen balance studies carried out using healthy *young men* many years ago. Amino acids are nitrogen-containing molecules. As they are metabolized, the nitrogen is excreted. By measuring nitrogen loss (in urine, skin, hair, etc) and comparing it to nitrogen intake (as protein in food), researchers can arrive at Nitrogen Balance, where Nitrogen In = Nitrogen Out and calculate the protein intake that results in Balance.

But recent research suggests this method does not account for all uses of amino acids, and does not account for the effects of aging on muscle loss. The concept of nitrogen balance refers to a minimum intake, not to an ideal or optimal intake for the needs of older adults.

Proposed increases in protein intake for older adults amount to an intake that is 50% or more above the current recommendation. Let's look at that 150 lb women again. Her conventional requirement for protein is 55 grams/day. One of the intake suggestions for older adults is 1.2 grams/kg/day, resulting in a daily intake of 80 grams protein. A 2017 study published in the British Journal of Sports Medicine suggests that a level of 1.6 grams/kg/day (0.73 grams per pound per day) significantly improves muscle mass and strength in response to resistance exercise training. That calculates to 110 grams of protein per day for our sample woman, if she is in a training program.

Furthermore, experts advise that protein be consumed in relatively equal amounts spread between 3 meals per day to maximize protein digestion and utilization. A study of protein intake in older adults compared intake throughout the day. For people whose protein intake was distributed evenly between meals – averaging around 18-23 grams per meal -- muscle mass was higher, even if total daily protein intake was the same.

According to the grams/kg recommendations above, our sample woman would be eating about 25 grams of protein per meal, in line with the findings of that study. Intakes above 30 grams per meal provide no additional benefit to muscles. At higher total protein intakes, you should consider high protein snacks. The main take-away: lumping most of your protein into one big evening meal is not a great plan for muscle strength.

For some meals, particularly the evening meal, high protein is par for the course. Meals may be structured around a high protein entrée. A chicken breast or 4-5 oz burger will have close to 30 grams of protein, and that's not counting protein from the other foods, or second helpings.

Breakfast might be the most problematic when it comes to high protein. Many people eat little breakfast, and stick to higher carbohydrate foods like toast or oatmeal. Protein foods like milk or yogurt may be consumed, but you'd need 3-4 cups of yogurt to equal the recommended protein. Just thinking about that much yogurt at one meal sounds unappetizing.

One solution would be eggs, particularly omelets. A 2-egg omelet with an ounce of grated cheese would have around 22 grams protein. Add a piece of toast and the total protein in the meal is close to the recommended amount. The problem would be keeping that up day after day. Omelets could become boring, not to mention not always convenient or appealing.

You could try smoothies, using Greek style yogurt, which is high protein, blended with juice and fruit. Again this will be a very filling smoothie. Another option: smoked salmon (or other smoked fish). A half bagel topped with smoked salmon would pack a protein punch.

You could also adopt the habit of Second Breakfast (or Elevenses) if you get up very early. Have one modest breakfast early, have a second breakfast between 10 and 11. Both breakfasts should include about 12-15 grams protein from foods such as:

Yogurt
Milk
Eggs
Cheese
Peanut butter (or other nut butter)
Meat, fish, poultry
Beans
Nuts

Leucine may be your friend

So you're on board with eating more protein, and spreading your protein foods throughout the day. Is there anything more? Yes possibly. There's leucine.

Leucine is one of the essential amino acids. Research shows that it facilitates muscle growth by activating and controlling gene signals. It's interesting to note that, in human breast milk, leucine is the essential amino acid at highest concentration. It's unique muscle building effect would make sense, since human babies grow at a very fast pace during the months after birth.

In fact, the leucine content of protein of an adult's meal determines the muscle building impact of that meal. Muscle synthesis peaks 60-90 minutes after a meal. But aging is associated with resistance to muscle synthesis after meals. Leucine and higher protein intake can overcome this. There are studies of sedentary older adults showing that leucine content of a meal needs to be more than 1.8 grams to stimulate muscle synthesis.

Where can you find leucine? High protein foods like meat and eggs will be some of the best choices.

- 3 ounces of cooked turkey breast meat has over 2 grams
- 4 ounces of cooked lean beef has about 4 grams of leucine
- 1 oz of cheese (about ¼ cup grated) has about 1 gram
- 4 oz cooked chicken has 3.2 grams
- ½ cup dry roast soy beans has 1.5 grams
- ½ cup peanuts has 1.3 grams
- 1 cup cooked beans has about 1.2 grams
- 1 7-oz container low fat Greek yogurt has 1 gram
- 1 cup low fat milk or plain yogurt has about 0.8 gram
- 1 egg has .5 grams

So in general, meats and fish are good sources; a 4 oz serving has between 2 and 4 grams of leucine in addition to other protein. Cheeses have about 1 gram per ounce. Dairy foods have 1 gram or less per serving. Cooked legumes are another decent source.

As the understanding of leucine's unique role in muscle protein synthesis grows, body-building food products fortified with leucine, as well as leucine supplements, show up on store shelves. Some studies have been done on muscle synthesis, giving older people leucine supplements, with mixed results.

The key point should be this: leucine is an essential amino acid found in food. It has unique effects on muscle protein synthesis. However, leucine alone cannot create muscle protein. All other amino acids are necessary, and you can find those in high protein foods along with leucine. So just consume those foods. Eat high protein foods in roughly the same quantity at 3 or 4 meals/day, spread evenly throughout the day. Unless future research shows otherwise, taking separate leucine supplements on top of eating high protein foods is not likely to provide additional benefit.

The bad news is that sarcopenia is linked to aging and can lead to increasing immobility and weakness. The good news is that the health community now recognizes that sarcopenia can be diagnosed, and steps can be taken to minimize or perhaps reverse the impact and progression of the problem.

The other good news is that you are a very big part of the solution. And you don't need an official diagnosis to take control. A higher protein diet combined with training, particularly resistance training using weights and machines, perhaps directed by a competent trainer, are the two keys to combating the effects of sarcopenia.

7 ENERGY

The word "energy" conjures many important concepts. You might think of energy as stamina – the ability to keep running 5 miles a day at the same pace indefinitely. Or as mental energy, to wake up in the morning refreshed, ready to face the day, deal with whatever and enjoy life. You might feel you lack energy if you find you haven't slept well and need a nap. Or your mental energy might be drained by the thought of an unpleasant task you've been putting off.

Energy is mental and physical. Physical vitality can help you deal with the mental challenges. Mental fortitude can push you to find the physical energy to finish a difficult hike or get through a demanding physical therapy session after an injury. The point is: it's hard to pinpoint one thing that is "energy", and that can be fixed by diet or nutrition.

We'd like to think that aging shouldn't affect our energy level if we maintain a healthy weight and stick to an exercise plan. But as years go by, we realize we can't jog or walk or swim or bike as far or as fast as we could at 30. We tire more easily or we just go at a slower pace. It's as if we've morphed from the proverbial hare to the tortoise. But slow and steady still works fine in most situations. I see it as adjusting to a new way of enjoying so many activities, and not pushing oneself in ways that are just not realistic. If hiking up a trail that used to take an hour now takes 1-1/2 hours, well so be it. You still get to the top of the trail and enjoy the view.

Energy 101

In a strictly metabolic sense, the energy your muscles and brain use for fuel is calories. Thanks to the diet industry, you may think of calories as something bad, to be avoided. But without calories, you're dead. Sorry to be blunt, but calories are to you as gasoline is to your car. Without them you go nowhere.

Everyone has what's called a basal energy (calorie) requirement. That's the number of calories needed daily just to support life. That number depends on your age, weight, muscle mass and gender. For most older women, the number is in the 1100-1300 calorie range.

If you spent the day lying in bed, you'd need that basal amount of calories just to breathe, think, have a heart beat, etc. On top of that, if you eat food you need a few more calories to run digestion. It's sort of like the amount of gasoline a car burns while idling. The car may not be moving, but it's burning gas if it's sitting in traffic or at a stop light.

Of course the car burns more gas as it starts to move, and you burn more calories when you move. How many you burn for activity depends on your fitness level, muscle mass, the activity, length of activity, weight and gender. For the average person, most calories are used for your basal requirement plus digestion.

Measuring Calorie Expenditure

The Metabolic Equivalent of Task (MET) list includes dozens of activities, many divided into different levels of exertion. Each activity has a value. For example, sitting quietly has a value of 1. Slow walking on level ground has a value of 2. Running a 10 minute mile has a value of 9.8. An MET calculator uses your weight, time spent at the activity and the MET value to compute the number of calories used.

According to the MET calculator, a woman who weighs 150 lbs would burn about 68 calories sitting for an hour. She'd burn 136 walking slowly for an hour, and 668 running at a 10 minute mile pace for 60 minutes. Keep in mind, in order to burn 668 calories, she must maintain that pace for the full 60 minutes, no slowing down. If you're interested in doing some of your own MET calculations, check the links in the general reference section for MET lists and handy online calculators.

The food you eat from one meal to the next can provide energy for immediate needs. You eat breakfast, you go out for a walk, and at least some of the breakfast food fuels your walk. The carbohydrates from foods like bread, cereal, potatoes or fruit are digested and absorbed as glucose, which fuels muscle activity. Fat is also used for fuel, but it's not the preferred fuel.

If you eat nothing before your walk, you might find yourself lagging during the walk. You can still keep walking though, because you have energy stores to cover short- and long-term deficits. Short term needs are covered by glycogen, a storage form of carbohydrate, which can be mobilized quickly to maintain blood glucose levels and fuel muscle movement.

After glycogen is used up (that's a long walk), fat may be used for an larger portion of your energy needs. On a gram for gram basis, fat has more than twice the calories (9) of carbohydrates (4), so it's a more concentrated fuel. In more extreme situations, protein from muscle and other tissues is broken down into amino acids, which are converted to glucose and then used for fuel. This is why drastic diets and starvation lead to loss of muscle tissue along with fat. Glucose is the preferred energy source for brain cells, so your body will maintain blood glucose levels at the expense of muscle tissue.

So if glucose and fat are energy sources, why don't you feel more energetic if you eat more food? It's a fair question. Here's a good comparison: your car runs on gasoline. Does it go faster or farther if you dump buckets of gasoline over the hood? No. Your car can only use a requisite amount of gasoline at an one time for a given speed or distance.

Likewise, your body can only digest and metabolize food fuels at a certain rate. Blood sugar will only increase up to a level, at which point hormones are mobilized to clear excess out. If muscle cells aren't using it, excess is moved into fat cells. Muscle cells can only accept and process a set amount of glucose at one time. So loading up on food does not make you feel more energetic in the short term. Anyone who has overindulged at a holiday meal knows that excess food can have quite the opposite effect.

Why Am I Tired?

Even with sufficient calories on board, you can still feel tired or fatigued. Other than calorie deficit, there are numerous reasons for feeling tired or fatigued including:

- Medical conditions, such as low thyroid or heart disease
- Poor sleep
- Medication side effects
- Poorly controlled diabetes
- Dehydration
- Depression, stress or other psychological issues
- Excess use of alcohol or recreational drugs
- Delayed effect of extreme exertion
- Jet lag
- Hunger
- Anemia. While this may be a nutritional issue, any anemia needs to be diagnosed properly. You might be iron deficient due to unrecognized blood loss from a medical issue, not from poor iron intake.
- Chronic malabsorption of nutrients due to digestive disturbances, leading to nutrient deficiencies and impaired energy metabolism
- Lack of fitness
- Lack of exercise

The latter two might seem counterintuitive, but in fact as you age, you can lose fitness and muscle mass quickly if you're immobilized for a period of time. Lack of muscle mass and muscle fitness can make you feel fatigued when you do move. This is why it's so very important to follow rehab recommendations after an injury or illness, to get muscles moving and rebuild stamina.

Many of the other potential contributing factors are not

related to diet or nutrition, and may be out of your control. Certainly medical issues like diabetes, medication side effects and malabsorption syndromes need to be discussed with a physician and treated properly. Chronic sleep problems, anemia and depression should also be discussed. So what is under your control?

1. Fitness: as discussed above, staying active helps to maintain muscle mass and fitness and improve stamina
2. Dehydration: maintain adequate fluid intake, especially in hot weather or dry climates. Dehydration can make you feel fatigued.
3. A balanced diet with adequate protein at all meals, as discussed in the discussion of sarcopenia in Chapter 6.
4. Fuel adequately before physical activities.
5. Avoid excess alcohol and recreational drugs
6. Create a sleep environment that's conducive to *sleep*.
7. Take steps to build your nutrition status back up after any prolonged period of illness, malabsorption or unplanned weight loss.

Sleep

Everyone has an occasional night of poor sleep. You can resolve any lingering fatigue by sleeping well the next night. Chronic sleep disruption should be discussed with your medical provider. Medical problems, medications, snoring, sleep apnea and depression can all disrupt sleep.

There aren't any specific nutritional interventions for sleep. Obesity is a nutrition-related issue, and obesity can

I've heard anecdotes about sleep and supplements, so I'm passing this on as an FYI. Some people believe taking vitamins, such as multiples or B vitamins, in the evening before bedtime affects sleep in a negative way. I've also heard the suggestion that vitamin D taken in the evening disrupts sleep. There's no clinical evidence; there may not even be studies, so take this with a grain of salt lead to sleep disruption, as it's linked to sleep apnea and reflux disease. Whether you're obese or not, eating big meals shortly before bedtime can lead to poor sleep. Caffeine and alcohol can affect sleep cycles. Your ability to metabolize these chemicals can change with age, so you might not realize that your afternoon coffee or chai is contributing to worsening sleep difficulties. And don't discount other health halo foods and beverages with stimulant properties, such as chocolate and green tea.

Underfueling

Do you think like this: *I'll eat a tiny breakfast, just some toast, and go out for a walk or golf game or swim. Then I'll reward myself later for my exercise with a piece of pie. With ice cream!*

This is a common behavior of dieters everywhere. The thinking goes like this: *"I'm burning X number of calories, and if I don't eat beforehand I can eat back all those calories later as a treat."* Not a good plan for so many reasons.

Reason #1: you're exercising but don't have readily available energy. So your metabolism has to shift to a different fuel source. Your exercise/workout isn't as effective. You're more tired.

Reason #2: you burned calories earlier in the day. But your loading up on calories later, when you aren't doing very much. Your metabolism responds to excess calories by storing them away.

This isn't a good weight control strategy for anyone at any age. A few years ago, a study of young female swimmers noted that the girls who ate before training had more effective training sessions and had less body fat than the girls who ate nothing, and then ate back their calories later.

The point is, if physical activity is on the schedule, eating something beforehand helps prevent fatigue. You perform better and get more benefit from the exercise.

Hunger

Underfueling and hunger have a lot in common, although underfueling is more about the failure to eat ahead of physical activity. But both involve insufficient food intake. You can sit around all day and get hungry, if you don't eat for several hours. And lack of food can make you feel tired, draggy, headachy and cranky even if you've been sedentary.

Here's an example you can probably relate to: you're traveling by plane a long distance in one day, involving a close connection or two. You have no time to buy food at the connecting airports (or you don't want to spend the money) and of course there's precious little food on planes anymore. So unless you prepared in advance, packing snacks in your carry-on bag, you're going to be hungry. Traveling is stressful enough, and you'll have the added stress of not eating for hours. You'll arrive at your destination feeling exhausted, even though you spent the day sitting.

Malnutrition

Profound fatigue can result from compromised nutritional status. Intestinal dysfunction due to infections (C. difficile, E. coli, salmonella, parasites, listeria), chemotherapy or other diseases is one culprit. Prolonged poor food intake due to cancer, extreme stress, post-surgical recovery or loss of appetite is another culprit. You may experience a creeping sense of fatigue and listlessness, as well as unplanned weight loss.

The effects of poor nutrition can be exacerbated in older adults. Unexplained weight loss and loss of appetite are common. Unfortunately a significant proportion of that type of weight loss is muscle mass, making it harder to recover.

In order to restore your energy and sense of vitality, you have to build your diet back up. You need adequate calories and protein. Vitamins and minerals are essential for energy metabolism, so you need to focus on nutritionally dense foods and beverages. You'll find more detailed information on rebuilding your nutritional status in Chapter 14.

Energy Comes From Food

Strictly speaking, all foods and beverages that have calories provide energy. Products without calories provide no energy. Strangely, plenty of so-called energy boosting foods and beverages *have no calories.* One recent marketing campaign claims that a certain energy shot product has zero calories, but provides 5 hours of energy. Oh really?! Let's get back to our sample 150 lb women above. She will burn 68 calories an hour just sitting quietly. So 5 hours of sitting uses 340 calories. How does a zero calorie product supply 340 calories? It doesn't.

The marketing for so-called "energy" products capitalizes on consumers' generally poor understanding of what energy is. It's calories; fuel for our bodies. But marketers believe you'll confuse calories with stimulants. Energy products rely on caffeine and other stimulants. Some throw in a few B vitamins, as if vitamins alone magically produced energy. They do not. That's like saying spark plugs will make your car go, even in the absence of gasoline. Obviously false.

The best energy foods

So what foods are good for energy? It depends on whether you're looking for quick energy or sustained energy, or both. Quick energy would be important if you've been out hiking or biking or playing golf or tennis for a 2-3 hours and you need to keep going. Or perhaps you're running a marathon. In order to keep going, you need to eat or drink something with calories. In both of these situations, a food or snack that combines quick energy with more sustained energy is the best plan. Something with a bit of sweetness from sugar (quickly absorbed calories) along with starchy carbohydrates, which are digested slowly to glucose and kick in after the sugars are used. And of course it should be a food or beverage you like and that fits the situation.

A variety of foods fit that description, such as:

- Fresh fruit, such as bananas, oranges, grapes and plums
- Dried fruit,, such as raisins, apricots, pineapple
- Granola or snack bars
- Trail mix, with dried fruit, nuts and maybe granola
- Sandwich such as PB&J
- Crackers or pretzels

Or course, other foods you enjoy fit this description, such as cookies, pastries, muffins and candy. When you need quick energy during physical activity, these can work well as fast fuel. They are not the ideal choice if you need an afternoon snack because you're hungry. In those situations, more substantial foods are better choices. Small sandwiches, cheese and crackers, hummus and vegetables, fresh fruit and yogurt, dried fruit and nuts – these are all examples of snacks that provide calories in a more sustained form, digested and absorbed more slowly than sweets.

Think of it as your energy *diet*

Rather than focus on certain foods as ideal energy sources, focus on your whole diet. Your diet can make you feel draggy and tired, or it can make you feel energized. Adding energy foods to a junky diet isn't going to help. Ideally your whole diet creates energy harmony. Which would not mean you never, ever feel tired or fatigued. Rather, it means diet and food are rarely contributing factors.

So what kind of diet is that? It's a diet that makes sustained energy available throughout the day. How do you achieve that?

1. 3-4 modest meals or meals and snacks spread roughly evenly during the day
2. Meals/snacks include high protein foods to moderate the speed of digestion.
3. You avoid high sugar meals/snacks, *unless* you need a snack for quick energy during physical activity.

Even then, it's better if your quick energy snack includes starchy carbs and/or fat so the energy flow is sustained.

4. The first meal of the day includes significant protein, along with carb foods for energy, as well as healthy fats

Enough with the generalities. Here are some examples of a day's worth of energy:

Day 1

First meal
2 eggs (soft boiled or poached, or scrambled in small am't olive oil or on non-stick pan)
2 pieces of toast or English muffin (good with poached eggs)
Juice or some fresh fruit (berries, melon, orange, grapefruit)

Second meal
Wrap made with large tortilla (or flat bread), grated cheese, leftover cooked chicken pieces, chopped tomatoes/cucumbers/peppers/grated carrot/lettuce/spinach/etc, salsa or other flavored sauce
½ cup berries mixed with vanilla Greek style yogurt

Third meal/snack
At home: whole grain crackers, cheese slices or nut butter, raw carrots
Meeting friends for coffee: latte, scone or muffin
Meeting friends for happy hour: cheese, olives, flat bread, wine

Fourth meal
Grilled meat or fish of your choice
Seasoning of your choice, or prepared sauce
Grilled vegetables
Grilled potatoes or corn, or bread or rice (optional, if not worried about dieting for weight loss)

Day 2

First meal
Oatmeal with dried fruit, chopped nuts, sprinkle of wheat germ, topped with milk/vanilla or honey yogurt

Second meal
Tossed green salad with cheese and/or nuts and/or cooked meat or fish, large variety of fresh vegetables, olive oil vinaigrette
Bread/pita/flat bread/whole grain crackers/muffin

Third meal/snack
Vegetable style soup with grated cheese

Fourth meal
Broiled/grilled or pan fried meat of choice (could be burger)
Bread/bun/potato
Sautéed vegetables or tossed green salad

Day 3

First meal
bowl of low fat yogurt/Greek style yogurt
juice or fresh fruit
½ toasted bagel

Second meal
Leftover cheese vegetable pizza

Third meal/snack
Apple or banana
Peanuts or cashews

Fourth meal
Soft tacos with refried beans, grated cheese, cooked ground beef, salsa, chopped tomatoes, chopped lettuce

Of course, days don't always go as planned when it comes to food. The examples are rather idealized, but the point is to show you what a normal day of energy-sustaining food can look like. Calories and protein are spread evenly throughout the day, derived from whole foods in modest portions. By contrast, here's what an energy-sustaining day does *not* look like:

Bad Day

First meal
Sugar-sweetened latte
Donut

Second meal
French fries
Soft drink

Third meal/snack
Sugar sweetened iced coffee
Super-sized chocolate chip cookie

Third and ½ meal/snack
Beer
Plate of nachos

Fourth meal
Pasta Alfredo
Bottomless bread basket
Small tossed salad with blue cheese dressing
Red wine

Fourth and ½ meal/snack
Bowl of ice cream

Why this a bad day?

- Most of the food intake is shifted to late in the day
- Heavy on processed food, fat and sodium
- Almost all of the protein is late in the day, and there's not enough of it in general
- Too many simple sugar meals/snacks, metabolized quickly for sustained energy, probably leaving you hungry and dragging.
- Looks like excess calories
- Where are the vegetables and fruit?

So not a good example of an energy-sustaining meal plan. Energy-draining is more like it. And there's another fatigue-inducing problem: so much food eaten late in the day can disrupt sleep, causing you to feel tired the next day.

Ideally the majority of your days should resemble the first 3 examples. In which case, you can deal with the occasional day or two of dietary disruption and then get back on track.

Fatigue is a complex problem with many potential causes, some of which are related to nutrition and diet. If I had to rank the top 5 dietary factors that contribute most to garden-variety fatigue complaints, the list would look like this:

1. Inadequate food early in the day; food intake skewed to late in the day
2. Meals or snacks that contain too much sugar
3. Inadequate fueling for physical activities
4. Too much reliance on stimulants like caffeine in place of food.
5. Dehydration

As we age, energy and stamina will wane, but you can be proactive and take steps to minimize the impact. Your best defense is to address any medical or sleep problems and make sure your diet is energy-friendly.

8 DIGESTION AND FIBER

The digestive system might be the one body function you think about at some point every day. It's hard not to. Digestion events happen throughout the day: you eat, you drink, you eliminate, you might feel hunger or satiety, bloating or gas, gurgling or acid reflux. Or your stomach and intestines might not bother you at all, which in itself is an event.

The digestive system has lots of moving parts. To describe it as complicated is an understatement. Here are a few fun facts I picked up from the online course "Integrative and Functional Nutrition'" from the Academy of Nutrition and Dietetics:

- The digestive system has 10 times more cells that the rest of your body.
- There are more neurons in the digestive system than in the spinal cord or the nervous system that runs throughout your body
- The digestive system produces ¾ of the neurotransmitters in your body, including 95% of the serotonin
- 70-80% of your immune system is in the gut
- 100 trillion bacteria, more than 500 species

Recently our understanding of gut function has become much more sophisticated. It's not just about the moving parts – chewing, swallowing, intestinal absorption -- it's also about those 100 trillion microbes. Our health – mental and physical –

may depend on what types of bacteria inhabit our intestines. Which bacteria are beneficial and how do we encourage them? We don't have all those answers yet.

This chapter will cover current information about the nutrition-digestion connection, as well as emerging information about the digestion-health connection. Before launching into that exciting stuff, let's briefly review the digestive system.

Digestion 101

There is no nutrition without digestion. Digestion is the process of breaking down the food we eat into components that can be absorbed into blood and transported to tissues. The process involves mechanical (chewing), chemical (stomach acid) and biochemical (enzymes, transport molecules) activity. Now we know it also involves microbiological activity (gut microbes).

Digestion starts in the mouth, where food is chewed and mixed with saliva, which initiates digestion of carbohydrates. Food travels down the esophagus to the stomach, where it's mixed with hydrochloric acid, which initiates digestion of proteins.

After some time in the stomach, food is released slowly through a duct into the upper small intestine, where enzymes that digest fats, carbohydrates and proteins take over. The small intestine is divided into 3 sections: duodenum, jejunum and ileum. As food travels through these sections, nutrients are absorbed; some nutrients are absorbed only in specific regions.

What is not broken down by digestion and absorbed then moves into the large intestine, where gut microbes may ferment certain of the leftover substances. Eventually the unused remains of your food are eliminated as poop. Well, the official term would be feces.

This is all very straightforward, but as we all know so many things can go wrong:

- Diarrhea – infection, bad food
- Stomach or gas pain – bad food, infection, medical condition
- Constipation – poor diet or a medical issue
- Stomach ulcers
- Reflux
- Mouth sores
- Chewing problems due to tooth problems
- Bloating
- Cancers of the digestive system
- Malabsorption diseases such as Crohn's or irritable bowel disease

Unfortunately, as we age these problems seem to come along more frequently or hang around longer. The pharmaceutical industry has taken note. Medications for reflux or acid stomach are big sellers. We are all urged to get regular colonoscopies, which actually is one medical procedure that can *prevent* a dire disease.

Fixing digestive complaints with food or nutrition interventions is a very compelling idea. And in fact many problems are directly or indirectly impacted by what we eat, and can be ameliorated with dietary changes. But some issues can't be fixed by diet alone. If you're struggling with symptoms that are not improving, medical attention is recommended.

Fiber

In the nutrition universe, fiber and digestion go hand in hand. What was once dismissed as "roughage" in the early 20th century rose to prominence in the 1970's, as research linked high fiber diets especially to decreased risk of various diseases. Fiber became a kind of universal super-food. People bought bags of wheat bran and sprinkled it on everything to boost fiber intake, which was supposed to solve all kinds of problems, constipation being the most prominent.

But what exactly is fiber? When researchers started to analyze food, they found that the indigestible parts of food -- "fiber" – includes a wide variety of substances with different potential health effects. Here's the official definition:

"non-digestible soluble and insoluble carbohydrates (with 3 or more monomeric units), and lignin that are intrinsic and intact in plants; isolated or synthetic non-digestible carbohydrates (with 3 or more monomeric units) determined by FDA to have physiological effects that are beneficial to human health."

In other words, not just wheat bran or the stringy parts of celery. Chemically speaking, food fiber can be a gum or gel or a chain of carbon units that cannot be broken apart by digestive enzymes. The molecular structure of a fiber determines its behavior in the gut.

The term soluble fiber refers to non-digestible carbohydrates that bind water, forming a viscous gel. These gels have important functional properties in the large intestine, including:

- Interference with bile acid reabsorption, which helps lower blood cholesterol levels. Foods high in soluble fiber – such as oats, beans, apples or psyllium seed -- are well known components of a cholesterol-lowering diet.
- Fermentation by colonic bacteria, producing short chain fatty acids. These unique fat molecules are thought to be important for the health of the cells lining your gut. While fermentation can produce gas, which might be annoying, it's an important symbiotic relationship. You eat fiber in foods; gut bacteria utilize that fiber for their own purposes; some of the byproducts are helpful to you.
- Laxative effect due to stool bulking

Insoluble fiber, found in foods like wheat bran or vegetable peels, doesn't bind water and form gels. These types of fiber are not known for a lipid lowering effect, but are important for laxation. In this case, the laxative effect is caused by the fiber directly irritating the lining of the gut, which leads to secretion of water and mucous into the large intestine, which increases fecal bulk.

This isn't meant to imply that one type of fiber is "better" or "healthier" than another. Plant foods are our natural fiber sources, and some plant foods are better sources of certain types of fiber than others. But most plant foods represent mixes of a variety of fiber types. If you think about how different plant foods are from each other – apples are nothing like grains are nothing like broccoli are nothing like lentils – it's easy to understand how fiber types will vary from one food to another.

Insoluble non-gel forming fibers are higher in foods like wheat bran, other whole grains and fruits and vegetables, especially the peels. Foods that are higher in soluble gel-forming fibers include:

Oats
Legumes
Apples, pears, oranges, apricots
Prunes (dried plums)
Psyllium seed
Flax seed

How much fiber?

Various government and public health agencies make recommendations for fiber intake. Why? Because years of research indicates that higher fiber diets are linked to health benefits, including:

- Weight control: fiber is filling, giving a feeling of satiety so you eat less.
- Normalization of bowel movements: fiber is a well known remedy for constipation, but certain fiber can help with diarrhea thanks to its effect on gut bacteria and colon function.
- Lowering blood cholesterol (soluble fiber)

- Helps control blood sugar (soluble fiber)
- Encouraging healthy gut microbes.

The US Dietary Guidelines suggest 14 grams dietary fiber per 1000 calories eaten per day. In other words, if you typically eat about 1500 calories, you'd aim to get 21 grams of fiber. The Daily Value recommendation for total fiber intake is 25 grams for a person eating 2000 calorie/day. This is the number used on the Nutrition Facts panel on food labels. The label will state grams of total fiber per serving as well as % DV (% of 25 grams). A food with 5 grams of fiber per serving would represent 20% of DV.

The National Library of Medicine suggests 21-38 grams per day. The higher end of the range applies to adult men who eat more food. Meanwhile the National Fiber Council suggests 32 grams per day. So in general, the ballpark figure of 14 grams per 1000 calories is on target.

None of these recommendations distinguish between soluble and insoluble fiber types. The National Cholesterol Education Program recommends 20-30 grams of fiber/day, of which 10-25 grams should be *soluble* fiber to lower LDL cholesterol. This recommendation is based on research showing that soluble, gel-forming, fiber can help lower cholesterol when consumed at a certain level.

How does that soluble fiber recommendation translate to food? Here are some examples:

- ¾ c up of dry oats has about 3 grams; that's about 1-1/2 cups cooked oats.
- A cup of cooked beans has 4-5 grams.
- An orange has about 2 grams.
- A cup of Brussels sprouts has about 4 grams

So in order to get to 10 grams soluble fiber, you'd have to eat significant amounts of these types of foods every single day.

These are just some examples of foods that are particularly high in soluble (gel-forming) fiber. Oats are perhaps the best known. But all high fiber foods are a mix of different types of fiber. And there are different forms of soluble and insoluble. Apples have pectin; oats have beta-glucan; both are gel-forming soluble fiber, but have very different molecular structures.

Because there are so many different types of fiber in high fiber foods, one person's digestive system might be affected differently from another's. Your helpful high fiber food might be your spouse's digestive nightmare. The point is this: while there are plenty of recommendations to eat more of certain fiber foods, one or more of those foods might not work for *you*. In which case, just find other options. The choice of plant foods is enormous.

Some good fiber sources are typically consumed as add-ins for other foods. Psyllium seed is used in popular laxative preparations, such as Metamucil, but you can also buy less processed psyllium husk or powder. One teaspoon of psyllium powder has an impressive 3 grams of total fiber, 1 gram of which is soluble. It can be added to smoothies or other foods where the gel-forming effect is not objectionable. Flax seed has 3 grams total fiber per tablespoon. Chia seed is another option, with about 5 grams per tablespoon. You probably wouldn't just chow down on plain flax or chia seeds, but they can be added to cooked cereal or a smoothie or a baked item like muffins or bread. Thanks to its gel-forming properties, chia can be used to make pudding. Likewise, wheat bran can be purchased in bulk and added to cooked cereal or to recipes for breads or muffins.

Fiber supplements and additives

As noted above, fiber is defined as non-digestible carbohydrates. These types of carbohydrates come in many forms. The function of any one depends on its chemical structure. There is plenty of stuff in food that can technically be described as "fiber", since it fits the non-digestible definition. But that doesn't necessarily mean it's *functional*. In other words, just because it's non-digestible doesn't mean it has a recognizable health benefit. Non-digestible carbohydrates are not all created equal.

This is an important concept to understand when it comes to fiber. Food manufacturers are adding ingredients that technically fit the definition of fiber to processed foods for marketing purposes. Problem is, some of this stuff has no recognizable *function*. And when it comes to fiber, function is key.

Fiber supplements and fiber additives are typically non-digestible carbohydrates extracted from a plant source, and added to a food like yogurt or ready-to-eat cereal or an energy bar. Some powdered fiber supplements can be mixed into your morning coffee. Ideally from a manufacturing point of view, these have no affect on flavor or texture; they disappear into the food, but are featured prominently on the package label: "High Fiber!!" "Contains _X_ grams fiber!!" And technically those claims are true. The yogurt or processed cereal has X grams of non-digestible stuff. The consumer thinks "Great! I don't need to eat vegetables. I can eat yogurt."

Unfortunately, that "fiber" might not be doing much for your health. Popular fiber additives like inulin and wheat dextrin, fit this description. They can be fermented by bacteria in the colon, but that fermentation means they do not form highly viscous gels, important for functions like increasing stool bulk or lowering cholesterol. Suffice it to say, the best sources of functional fibers, that impact laxation, cholesterol, blood sugar and gut health are intact high fiber foods.

If you use some of these fiber supplement products and feel they are helpful, I'm not going to argue with your experience. But no amount of fiber additives or fiber tablets can substitute for the fiber in whole foods. A plant-based diet of whole foods contains a mix of many types of fiber, far preferable to a daily dose of one single type.

Assessing your intake

How much fiber are we actually eating? Diet surveys show that in the US, most adults get a total of only 10-15 grams/day, about half of the recommended intake. This isn't surprising, as surveys consistently show that very few people eat the recommended servings of vegetables, fruits and whole grains, which are the primary sources of fiber.

What about you? If you track your nutrient intake with a food/calorie tracker, you might sometimes wonder about your fiber totals. You feel you're eating plenty of high fiber foods, but your numbers seem low. Many foods in these databases are missing data on several nutrients, fiber being one of them. You might be eating plenty of fiber, but your totals are not accurate because when the fiber column has no data, it's entered as zero.

The easiest low tech way to monitor fiber intake is to eat a diet that's primarily plant-based. There are plenty of other benefits to this type of diet; it's the diet of choice for prevention of numerous chronic diseases, and is helpful for weight management.

Are you getting 20 grams? 22 grams? Relax. Rather than adding up grams of fiber, think about it in terms of the volume of plant foods on your plate. Here are some general guidelines:

1. A day's worth of food should be about 75% plant-sourced foods. In other words, if all your food was on a plate, about ¾ of the food on that plate would be plant-based.
2. Most of that volume would be fruit and/or vegetables
3. Fresh fruit and vegetables are preferable, although obviously some vegetables cannot be eaten raw (potatoes, winter squash, etc). Frozen and canned fruit and vegetables are good substitutes.
4. Whole grain foods are preferred, especially when that choice makes a difference. Example: you eat lots of bread, in which case choosing more whole grain breads increases overall fiber intake. But if you only eat pancakes once or twice a year, and don't care for whole grain versions, why bother?
5. If you feel you still need a fiber boost, adding small amounts of flax or chia seeds or psyllium powder to other foods can help.

Think about a bowl of cereal. Most of the volume in the bowl should be cereal (perhaps granola or bran cereal or shredded wheat), plus some fruit (such as fresh berries, banana or raisins), topped off with some milk or yogurt.

A stir fry for dinner is another good illustration. Stir fry lots of vegetables, add a small amount of chicken, pork, beef, tofu or fish, and serve over rice. If you use tofu, your whole meal is plant based.

How about a bean chili. Make the chili with beans, tomatoes, peppers and onions. Serve with rice or tortillas or cornbread. If you add a modest of amount of cooked meat, the meal is still primarily plant-based.

This model works for more traditional-looking meals as well. The key is to reduce the portion size of meat or chicken or fish and leave more room on your plate for plant foods. A modest 4-oz piece of chicken can be accompanied by larger portions of potatoes and broccoli. Or leave out potatoes and have two different vegetables, perhaps spicy green beans and roasted Brussels sprouts.

What about…..

Poop. Constipation and diarrhea might be the main reasons people think about fiber in the first place. Fiber has long been promoted as a solution for constipation, but how much and what kinds? As you can see, it's not just about bulking up on "fiber"; there are so many variations and they work in different ways to promote stool bulk and laxation.

The best solution would be a mix of all those fiber-filled plant foods everyday. Gel-forming fibers relieve constipation by holding water and increasing stool bulk. Insoluble fibers cause colon cells to secrete water and mucous, which also has a laxative effect.

How much? Which foods? That's up to you. One person's solution – whether oatmeal or spinach or kidney beans or prunes – might be another's digestive nightmare. At this point in your life, you probably have some idea about foods that don't agree with you. Short of some drastic life-changing event, you should go with what you know, increasing the high fiber foods that work for you, if necessary.

Diarrhea is a rather non-intuitive reason to think about

fiber. Many people assume fiber makes it worse, but that's not always the case. Soluble fiber can help, by holding water in stool; psyllium fiber is a known treatment for chronic diarrhea. Of course, the cause of diarrhea should be identified and treated, especially in the case of an infection. But sometimes, after an infection or medical condition has been cleared, the diarrhea remains, and soluble fiber might help.

My Fiber Plan

I have no idea how many grams of fiber I'm eating day to day, and I don't care. I try to include variety every day, but my clear preference is vegetables, followed by fresh fruit. I do not take fiber supplements and I do not buy processed foods fortified with fiber ingredients.

And contrary to what one might expect from a nutrition professional, I'm not a big fan of whole grain versions of certain foods, such as pasta. If whole grain breads or muffins makes sense from a taste standpoint, fine. Nothing like a crusty chewy artisanal whole grain loaf. But I'm not interested in minor increases in fiber from whole grain spaghetti or pie crust or pizza dough. I personally don't like how the flavor and texture are affected in those types of foods when whole wheat flour is substituted.

Here is how I rank high fiber foods according to their Bang for the Buck for taste, convenience, nutrition and versatility:

1. Vegetables: always available, wide variety of flavors and fiber types, nutrient dense, frequently low calorie, amenable to lots of different cooking and serving techniques, from tossed salad to roasted or grilled or highly seasoned cooked versions
2. Fresh fruit: doesn't need much preparation, refreshing, delicious in season, wide variety of fiber types, fuss-free, loaded with nutrients. Only drawback is that fruit not in season can be tasteless and pricey.
3. Frozen fruit or vegetables: a reasonable alternative

for out of season fruit and quick preparation vegetables.

4. Cooked legumes (beans): high protein plant foods, high fiber, great source of many other nutrients, useful in lots of different foods, from chili to soups to Mexican or Indian dishes to salads. Buy canned for extremely easy preparation.

5. Whole grains: cooked grains, such as oatmeal, brown rice, barley, etc can be used as breakfast cereal, casseroles, in soups, as a side dish or in grain-based salads. Certain high fiber ready-to-eat cereals – bran flakes, shredded wheat, etc -- fall into this category, too.

6. Whole grain flours: useful for breads, muffins, pancakes or quick breads. Can be used for cakes, pastries, cookies etc, but will impact flavor and texture while contributing little to overall fiber intake (OR: if you eat so many cookies that making them with whole wheat flour impacts your fiber intake, your diet needs re-thinking).

7. Dried fruit still has the original fruit's fiber content, but much more concentrated, because much of the moisture has been removed. If you eat significant amounts of dried fruit for the fiber – prunes come to mind – it's a good idea to consume some extra fluid. Keep in mind, dried fruit ends up being higher calorie per volume compared to the original fresh fruit version.

8. Whole grain versions of traditional foods: pasta, pizza dough, etc. Your choice.

9. Specialty ingredients like wheat bran, flax seed or chia seed. These do have lots of fiber, but typically they are used as mix-ins or toppings, not consumed in large amounts. I can't imagine anyone eat a big bowl of plain wheat bran or chia seed.

10. Nuts are plant foods and do have fiber, but they're also high fat and high calorie. Trying to boost fiber intake by eating nuts will significantly boost your

calorie intake. Unless that is your goal, you might rather think of nuts as nice additions to other plant-based foods, like salads or wraps or casseroles.

9 GUT MICROBES AND DIGESTIVE HEALTH

If fiber was the 20th century solution for digestive health, the 21st century is all about probiotics, otherwise known as gut bacteria, or the microbiota. The term microbiome refers to the genetic make up of the gut microbe population. Researchers use gene technology now to identify which microbes populate the gut, and so frequently speak of the "gut microbiome". Whatever term you use, it's about the bewildering mix of microorganisms living in our digestive systems.

When I told some acquaintances I was writing this book, one of them asked if I "believed in gut microbes." Which sounds silly; there isn't much to believe, since they're a fact of life. But I know what she meant: did I ascribe to new revelations about the importance of gut microbe populations to health. Yes I absolutely do.

As noted above, there are upwards of 100 *trillion* microorganisms, primarily bacteria, in the human gut. Here's another sobering thought: 90% of the cells in our bodies are microbes. Our own human cells are just 10%. Research has identified from 1000 to almost 1200 bacterial species that could inhabit the human digestive system. Your microbiome is affected by:

- Age: For example, infants have very different gut microbes than adults.
- General health and medication usage, especially antibiotics
- Where you live, which can affect types of bacteria in your gut as well as the diversity of types
- Your diet

Of all possible factors that can impact gut bacteria, diet is hugely important. Studies comparing the effects of different diet styles on gut microbes show that bacterial populations can shift significantly after less than a week of changing one's diet pattern, such as from meat-based to plant-based.

Diet works two key ways:

1. The food you eat encourages certain types of bacteria and discourages others, because gut bacteria live off the non-digestible components of the food you eat.
2. Microbes in food and beverages can impact your microbiome, if only temporarily. Fermented foods, from yogurt to craft beer, contain the microorganisms that created the food, which can colonize your gut. Other food may contain microorganisms because the food wasn't washed thoroughly or is slightly "off". Sometimes poorly cooked or washed food causes serious infections. But sometimes it's not a problem.

When it comes to the relationship between aging and the gut, there are two important questions:

1. Does aging itself impact the mix of gut microbes, and is that impact detrimental?
2. Can a healthy gut microbe population impact the aging process in a way that's beneficial?

In fact, some of the very earliest interest in gut microbes was inspired by an interest in prolonging life with fermented foods. Elie Metchnikoff, who won a Nobel Prize for his late 19th century work on immunology, noticed that long-lived people consumed more lactic acid producing bacteria in food, such as yogurt. In 1907, he wrote the original pro-probiotic book: "The Prolongation of Life" about his theories on aging and gut microbes, inspired by long-lived Eastern Europeans who eat a lot of yogurt. You may remember yogurt commercials on TV in the 1970's that used this longevity concept to sell yogurt.

So what is the effect of aging? There doesn't seem to be an

isolated effect of aging itself on the gut, or at least not one that's recognized as being solely due to age. But, as food choices and diet change with age, those changes do affect gut microbes. So the effect of age might really be about the effect of diet.

Unfortunately, aging may make diets increasingly limited and monotonous for a variety of commonplace reasons. Chewing difficulties, lack of interest in cooking, changing taste preferences and reliance on convenience foods means a more processed diet with fewer fiber-rich foods. A less diverse diet leads to less diversity in the gut microbiota. Certainly, increased use of medications can also impact gut microbes.

Microbes and aging

Can a healthy gut microbe population reverse, or lessen, adverse effects of aging? That's a very important question. The best information we have so far is from rodent studies, which provide some hints about how gut microbes might affect the aging process. For example:

- Germ-free mice have exaggerated responses to stress. Adding a strain of bifidobacteria to their guts normalizes their responses. Aging can reduce our ability to cope with stress in all its forms, so a healthy gut microbe population could help with that.
- The blood-brain barrier normally keeps unwanted molecules out of the brain. Aging leads to more permeability of this barrier, potentially contributing to brain dysfunction. Germ-free mice exhibit more permeable blood-brain barriers, but adding a strain of probiotic to their gut normalizes barrier function.

Because it contains 70-80% of your immune system, a healthy gut can improve your responses to inflammation and infections. There is evidence that risk for Type 2 diabetes, metabolic syndrome and some cancers is linked to characteristics of the gut microbiome. All of these diseases become increasingly common with age. Perhaps beneficial gut bacteria can decrease those risks.

Studies to clarify many of these potential impacts are on-going. Right now, at most, we can conclude that a healthy gut microbe population likely has a beneficial effect on some of the undesirable health aspects of aging, from immune function to brain function. Exactly how much of an impact, or more importantly, which bacteria provide the most benefit, are not known.

Probiotics

You've probably heard the term "probiotics", since it's a very hot topic in the media and in research. Probiotic refers to the microbes that take up residence in your intestines and confer a health benefit. Fermented foods are a major source of probiotics.

Humans have consumed fermented foods for thousands of years. Researchers speculate that early humans first developed a taste for alcohol by eating fermenting fruit. We continue to enjoy foods, such as beer, wine, alcoholic beverages, sauerkraut, aged cheese, dairy foods like yogurt and kefir, fermented soy foods and vegetables, and pickles. Many of these foods such as yogurt, kombucha, kefir and kimchi are gaining popularity beyond their traditional geographic locales.

Some fermented foods are believed to have medicinal properties. It makes some sense; humans have been eating these foods and many of the bacteria in those foods populate the human gut. Probiotic supplements, on the other hand, are a very new phenomenon. Manufacturers package mixtures of likely bacterial species into capsules and promote them for general health, weight loss and to relieve gastrointestinal symptoms.

Is the hype justified?

Considering all the hype, you'd think all the facts were in on the health benefits of probiotics. They are absolutely not.

We're just at the beginning of understanding some of the major issues, such as:

1. **Which bacteria live in the human gut?** At best, we have information about general groups (bacterial phyla), such as:
   - Firmicutes (includes Lactobacillus species)
   - Bacteriodetes
   - Actinobacteria
   - Proteobacteria

   Even then, the ratios of different bacterial groups to each other depends on factors like diet, geographic locale and genetics. According to The American Gut Project, some people have 90% Firmicutes and others have less than 1%. Why? And what, if any, are the health implications of that? To make it even more confusing, there are hundreds of possible species within each microbial phylum. Are they all equally beneficial?

2. **Which bacteria are beneficial, which are neutral, which might be harmful?** At the moment, we do not have good answers for any of those questions, although we do at least know about some microorganisms, such as salmonella or listeria, that cause acute infections. There's some general agreement about species that are likely beneficial, such as lactobacillus. But which lactobacillus? There are many varieties.

3. **Are there specific foods or diet that will predictably improve the health profile of your own gut bacteria?** We don't know for sure. A lot of the food recommendations are assumptions based on tradition. Yogurt, for example, has been consumed for centuries. People who eat yogurt seem to be healthy. Lactobacillus bacteria from yogurt can populate the gut; therefore lactobacillus species must be desirable.

It's important to understand these limitations, because many companies selling probiotic foods or supplements would like consumers to assume that anything with a probiotic Health Halo on the label is going to be beneficial.

Diet and gut microbes

Here's one thing we do know about the human gut: the population of bacteria can change pretty quickly in response to dietary changes. Research comparing plant-based vs. meat-centric diets has shown this quite clearly. Fundamentally different types of bacteria thrive when the host human eats lots of fiber-rich and carbohydrate-rich plant foods vs. a diet heavy on high fat and high protein animal-sourced foods like meat.

Suffice it to say your own gut microbe population will adapt and change in the short and long term if your diet changes. Think about how differently you might eat in summer (more fresh fruit and lighter foods) compared to winter (heavier foods, less fresh raw food, etc). Do you notice digestive function differences? How about when you travel to different countries and consume very different foods?

We also have some understanding about what all those trillions of gut bacteria are doing. A major function is fermentation/digestion of fiber, the various non-digestible carbohydrates discussed previously. Another important function is production of signaling molecules that impact metabolism or modulate inflammation. One potential effect of this is on obesity and weight management.

Research comparing the gut microbe populations in obese people vs. normal weight people finds consistent differences. And when obese people lose weight, their gut bacterial populations change to be more like normal weight people. Is this due to the changed diet, or some other effect of weight loss? Or, more intriguing, did the weight loss *diet* change the gut microbes, which in turn impacted metabolism, facilitating weight loss?

There is some evidence that certain gut microbe varieties are better at extracting energy from food and promoting fat storage that other microbes. So when you lose weight is it because of your diet, or is it because the gut microbe population changed in reaction to the diet?

We don't yet know the answer to this question. There's no evidence that this or that particular species of intestinal bacteria will cause or enhance weight loss. The general conclusion is that diet and gut microbes work together to influence weight. Research is trying to identify unique strains of microbes associated with weight loss.

Prebiotics

So-called prebiotics are specific food components that are fermented by those gut bacteria that we want to encourage. Eating foods with those non-digestible carbohydrates should lead to a healthy gut microbe population. That's the theory anyway.

Prebiotics are frequently promoted as something more special that just fiber. And certain specific forms of fiber are preferred by some gut microbes, so eating foods with those fiber types can give your gut bacteria an extra boost. For example, onions and Jerusalem artichokes are especially high in a carbohydrate called inulin, a fructo-oligosaccharide molecule, which is fermented by several varieties of microbe. So eating these foods encourages those types of bacteria.

Thanks to the marketing potential of inulin as a prebiotic fiber, it's now extracted from plant material and added to other foods, like yogurt or sports bars. The food label might brag "High Fiber!" or "contains prebiotics!". But inulin and some other prebiotics do not behave like the fibers that hold water or help with constipation or glucose control. So again, inulin is one kind of fiber, not the answer to all your fiber needs. Eating some foods with naturally occurring inulin is a nice idea. Relying on inulin-fortified snack bars or inulin tablets, not so much.

As if prebiotics weren't confusing enough, we can add the idea of "symbiotics" to the mix. This term isn't quite as popular for marketing purposes yet. Basically it means a food that contains probiotic bacteria plus prebiotic substances. A complete package of gut microbiota promotion. Exhibit A: yogurt. It contains both the beneficial bacteria plus the food those particular bacteria like to eat: lactose. Honestly, attaching a health-halo-techno-chemical name to something as simple and wholesome as yogurt is a bit much.

Better to just eat a variety of high fiber plant foods, so you consume a wide variety of fiber types. Plant foods contain other non-digestible carbohydrates that gut bacteria will ferment. In fact, instead of worrying about eating special prebiotics along with your probiotic foods, just eat a varied plant-based diet, and your fiber or prebiotic bases will be covered.

I personally never worry about prebiotics as a separate issue. I just eat plant foods, which contain natural prebiotics. It's much easier.

What is FODMAPS?

You may have heard the term FODMAPS in discussions of diet and digestive problems. FODMAPS stands for *"fermentable oligosaccharides, disaccharides, monosaccharides and polyols"*. These are carbohydrates and sugar alcohols that some people cannot digest properly, in which case gut microbes ferment them, causing a variety of digestive problems. While some of these substances, such as inulin, fit the official definition of fiber, some do not. Lactose (milk sugar), fructans (long chains of fructose molecules) and sugar alcohol low calorie sweeteners like sorbitol are FODMAPs molecules; some people cannot adequately metabolize them, but they are not fiber.

Low FODMAPs diets are frequently recommended for irritable bowel and similar chronic problems, but that doesn't mean these substances necessarily cause those conditions. Rather they might make them worse. Some people get relief on a FODMAPs diet; some do not. Some people may be sensitive to one type of FODMAP molecule, but not to others. Lactose is a good example; many people cannot digest lactose, and so avoid milk. But that doesn't mean they can't digest other FODMAPs type molecules.

One of the main problems with FODMAPs diets is that the list of foods to avoid is lengthy, causing extreme disruption to the diet. It's a shotgun approach: avoid almost everything; hopefully the problem food will be one of those.

Given all the publicity for this diet, it's surprising that there isn't a lot of good evidence that it consistently helps people with digestive symptoms, or that, if it does, the reason is elimination of a FODMAP substance.

Why try such a restrictive diet? If you've been dealing with chronic irritable bowel with no resolution, it could be helpful. But remember, it's a shotgun approach. If you do find relief on a FODMAPs diet, I suggest that at some point you investigate whether some of those foods might be added back with no trouble.

The Gut-Brain Axis

One of the most fascinating emerging fields in probiotic research focuses on the relationship between gut microbes and brain function. Obviously this would be extremely important for older people concerned about cognition and dementia.

You probably agree that, when you've had an intestinal infection -- feeling nauseous, bloated, perhaps with vomiting or diarrhea, and very uncomfortable – you were not in a happy mood. Or conversely, when you're stressed or anxious about a situation, your stomach or digestive system reacted badly, causing you more stress and discomfort? Have you ever used the phrase "gut instinct" to describe a decision or a feeling? How about "feeling butterflies in your stomach" when faced with an exciting or nerve-wracking situation? These are all examples of the gut-brain axis.

Gut-brain communication is not actually a new concept. It's the proposal that gut microbes direct the communication pathways that is new. The vagus nerve is the main path for this bi-directional communication between the digestive system and the brain. Neurotransmitters, including most of the serotonin, are made in the gut. It's estimated that the gut transmits nine times more messages to brain than the brain sends to the gut.

As mentioned above, the research so far has been done on animals, with provocative results. Behavior and brain chemistry can be altered by changing gut microbe populations. Memory and learning are impacted by different bacterial strains. Behavior that equates with depression in rodents is affected by gut bacteria. For example, germ-free mice – with no gut bacteria – react to stress situations in exaggerated ways compared to normal mice. If those mice are then given probiotics, their behavior normalizes.

Because this type of research depends on highly controlled environments and food, it's easy to study rodents. Not so easy to study humans. The effect of probiotic supplements or foods has been studied in healthy humans; in general there was a decrease in negative moods, with more improvement shown for people who started the study with more negative mood assessments. But not all studies showed consistent results.

Irritable bowel syndrome (IBS) is a frustrating and poorly understood affliction in which the gut-brain axis and the gut microbiota are disturbed. Inflammatory markers are elevated and IBS is typically accompanied by significant anxiety and depression. Some studies show reduction in depression when people with IBS are given probiotic supplements of specific strains of bacteria. The problem is that, when it comes to gut bacteria, there are *so many* potential strains to choose from. Perhaps 3 or 4 strains need to work together to resolve symptoms. If so, which ones? So far, optimism and anticipation of benefits outweigh solid evidence.

But that doesn't mean it isn't worth pursuing. It's certainly possible that at some time in the future, we can identify gut microbes that exert predictable effects on mood, anxiety or even certain mental illnesses. In which case probiotic foods or supplements and a diet that encourages growth of beneficial gut microbes might be part of treatment for certain psychological conditions.

Can you use this information right now to boost your mood with a specific probiotic? Not really. Probiotic supplements or foods marketed with mood-enhancing or stress-reducing messages are far, *far* ahead of the evidence. Which isn't to deny that you personally may feel better eating certain kinds of foods, or avoiding others. If yogurt or kombucha or kimchi calm your digestive system and therefore your mood, who's to argue? You recognize the benefit; that's what matters.

On The Research Horizon

Thanks to genetic technology, research on the gut microbiome can be done more easily and efficiently. And there is no lack of directions for this type of research.

Obesity is one area receiving a lot of attention. Gut microbe populations differ between lean and obese people. When obese people lose weight, their gut microbe population changes to be more like that of lean people. The key question is whether the weight loss or the weight loss diet causes that change.

There is some evidence that certain bacteria cause the human host to waste more energy, meaning it's not absorbed. The theory is that obese people have a microbiome that is the opposite, leading to more calorie absorption (or energy "harvesting").

Taking this idea one step further, some people have proposed fecal transplants as a weight loss strategy. Fecal transplants in mice show that when the microbiome of an obese mouse is transplanted into a germ-free mouse, that mouse gains more weight compared to mice implanted with lean-mouse microbes.

As yet, no one knows what a "lean" microbiome is exactly, exactly. Since gut microbe patterns differ around the world, and there are lean and obese people everywhere, there probably isn't just one effective lean microbiome. But identifying general characteristics of such a thing probably will happen. At which point we may have obesity treatments that involve probiotic foods or supplements or both.

Another important area of research focuses on immune function. Much of our immune system is in the gut, so it's conceivable that gut microbes can enhance immunity. But which ones are helpful and which ones are simply neutral, or cause inflammation. At some point we'll have more answers to these questions.

And farther down the research path, it may one day be possible to develop microbes that deliver drugs or nutrients, produced by specialized microbes. Instead of being prescribed an antibiotic you might be prescribed a particular probiotic mix of microbes that manufacture a natural antibiotic on site in your gut. We could have personalized microbe supplements for an individual's unique genetic profile: more of this nutrient, different metabolism of that nutrient, increased production of a signaling molecule, manufacture of a medication.

It's an exciting time for this type of research. We've come a long way since Elie Metchnikoff hatched his ideas about yogurt and longevity just over 100 years ago.

What to Do

Despite the lack of specific information on what is the healthiest and most beneficial gut microbiome, I think there's enough basic information to act on. After all, people have been eating fermented foods for a very long time.

One of the key take-aways from ongoing gut microbe research is that diversity is key. Focusing on just one strain of bacteria is the wrong strategy. Eating yogurt once and calling it a day is not going to do much for you. For the average person who wants to cultivate a healthy gut microbiome, I recommend both probiotic food and high fiber plant foods, daily, to encourage a diverse population of gut microbes to thrive.

What foods are those? For frequent or daily use, choose from some of these foods, popular for centuries around the world:

- Yogurt with active cultures
- Kefir
- Kombucha
- Miso soup
- Certain soft cheeses like gouda
- Fermented soy foods like tempeh
- Kimchi
- Sauerkraut
- Sour pickles (naturally fermented, not made with vinegar)

These foods are all very different from each other and harbor very different types of probiotics. Even yogurt and kefir – both made with milk – contain different types of bacteria. It's nice to try new foods, but if kimchi or kombucha aren't your thing, frequent yogurt is still helpful.

When I tried kombucha for the first time, I was surprised to find it has a nice light fizzy flavor. It's a lot like ginger beer – real ginger beer, not ginger ale – which is also a fermented probiotic drink, if you can find the real thing. Kimchi is an acquired taste, very strong flavored and used as a condiment. But it's a wildly popular dietary staple in Korea, so it must have something going for it.

Basically what I'm saying is keep an open mind. You might find that kombucha really agrees with you, or that kefir really isn't your thing, creating your own personal list of probiotic foods to enhance your health.

What do I do? Yogurt or kefir everyday, kombucha occasionally, sauerkraut and kimchi rarely. Other fermented foods when they're part of a meal. Along with a primarily plant-based diet, this works out just fine. I rarely need antibiotics, but if I've been taking them for a medical problem, I pay special attention to probiotic foods afterwards, to encourage re-colonization of healthy gut microbes. Again, the best approach includes probiotic foods like yogurt, kefir, kombucha, etc. along with a plant-centric diet, full of the fiber that beneficial bacteria prefer.

What about probiotic supplements?

Lack of solid evidence about which bacteria have beneficial effects on health hasn't stopped supplement manufacturers from jumping on the probiotic bandwagon. You can find plenty of probiotic supplements, containing various mixtures of bacterial species. Some foods never known for probiotic activity are now fortified with a fairy dusting of some sort of bacterial mix, just enough so the manufacturer can put a "Contains Probiotics!" health halo on the label.

Keep this in mind: there is *no standard definition* of a good or effective probiotic, so buyer beware. These are sold over-the-counter; the FDA only cares that such products are safe and contain what the label says, not that they are effective. Just because it says "probiotic" doesn't mean it's going to be beneficial.

Effective or not, probiotic supplements have two significant logistical problems:

1. Surviving stomach acid: the bacteria in the capsule do not live in your stomach. They have to make it to your intestines, preferably the large intestine, intact. Stomach acid can kill them off, so manufacturers have to devise a product that protects the microbes.
2. Viability: the bacteria has to be able to grow once you consume it. If they are not viable, you've wasted your money. Most have information about Colony Forming Units (CFU), or the number of bacterial cells in the supplement that can be expected to colonize your intestine. Many products need to be refrigerated to protect quality.

Supplement manufacturers and some food companies try to gain a marketing edge by touting unique strains of bacteria. For example, one yogurt company claims that the specific strain of bifidobacteria in its yogurt confers unique health benefits. Compared to all the other species in the bifidobacterium genus? How is this strain more beneficial? Or is it just equally helpful, but has a unique name that can be used as a selling point?

The difficulties of investigating which one out of dozens of strains of any bacteria species confer benefits are formidable. You can't create germ-free humans, as you can with mice, and then inoculate them with one bacteria and see what happens. We harbor trillions of gut microbes. Species populations vary and different species affect each others ability to thrive and multiply, or not. A human study proving benefits would have to go on for months or years in a controlled environment, with subjects eating an exacting diet and submitting to constant testing. Who would do that?

The best we have are educated guesses about bacterial groups that are likely beneficial. Supplements typically feature a select set of probiotics from those groups. But as noted above, there is no standard formula, and bacteria differ from one brand to another. Your friends might swear by one brand, but you don't see any effect or, worse, feel like it caused unpleasant problems. Doctors may recommend specific brands of probiotic supplements for conditions like irritable bowel syndrome, based on favorable experiences of other patients. Again, favorable experiences by other people do not guarantee that everyone will have a good outcome using a particular supplement.

I do not use probiotic supplements. Yet. I don't rule out the possibility that someday research will identify microbes that reduce cancer risk or help with weight management or improve cognition by way of the gut-brain axis. I'm always open to changing my mind if the evidence is strong. Until then, it's probiotic foods and a high fiber diet.

10 EYE HEALTH

For many of us, the first nutrition lessons was this: carrots were good for the eyes. Carrots are a good source of carotenes, beta carotene in particular. Carotenes are metabolized to vitamin A in the body, and in fact vitamin A is important for eye health. Years later, we know that nutrition for the eyes is vastly more complicated than that. Vitamin A is just piece of the puzzle when it comes to eye health.

Eye nutrition is a lifelong process. Some of the adverse changes in eyes that are associated with age started years before, from macular degeneration to dry eye syndrome to glaucoma to cataracts. There's an emerging body of evidence that some of these conditions are impacted by what we've been eating, or not eating. The key questions then are

What nutrients can help ward off serious eye problems?
Will diet changes at older ages have any beneficial effect?

Good research on the protective potential of diet would take years. Most of the information we do have is from studies looking at the effect of various nutrients on eye diseases of age. It puts an unfortunate slant on the results. Nutrition intervention is not going to cure existing eye diseases. It might slow progression. This doesn't sound very useful to the person with deteriorating sight.

Until there are better long term studies, the health establishment isn't going to promote nutrition as much as it could for to maintain eye health as we age. Which seems strange, since the structure and function of eyes depends on nutrients. And the supply of nutrients must constantly be renewed. Otherwise there would be no need to eat more carrots after that first nutrition lesson of childhood.

Eye structure and sight depend on all nutrients, just as all other tissues depend on all nutrients. But some are more critical to eyes, and recent research has helped to identify some of those:

- Omega-3 fats, particularly DHA, which is more concentrated in the eyes than any other tissue.
- Lutein and zeaxanthin, which are carotenes, and are concentrated in the macula
- Zinc, which is found in particularly high concentrations in the retina
- Vitamin A, which is essential for the numerous metabolic reactions that control vision. Beta-carotene and some other carotenes can be converted to the active form of vitamin A, and so can impact eye function.

Other nutrients that are known to be important for eye health include vitamin C, vitamin E and B2. But again, all nutrients play some in eye health and vision.

Dry Eye

When you visit an eye doctor for a check up, you're evaluated for several common age-related diseases, several of which have nutrition connections. Dry eye is typically not one of those, but maybe it should be.

Dry eye is a near but not-so-dear concern of mine. Several years ago, my eyes turned bright red, scratchy and even painful. So I kept splashing my eyes with water, not a good solution as I found out. The optometrist diagnosed Dry Eye, after doing a test that showed my eyes made no tears whatsoever. Zero. He had two solutions:

1. Constant moisturizing eye drops day after day, forever.
2. A surgery that plugged the holes in the eye lid that drained what little moisture I did have. I'd probably still need eye drops.

It sounded like my daily life would be dominated by eye drops every few hours, until he made an off-hand statement: "Some people say their eyes seemed better when they took flax." Bingo!

It was a 'eureka' moment. I knew immediately what that meant: omega-3 fats. This was back long before omega-3 fats were a household name with a major health halo. I'd read some about these special fats for professional reasons, but hadn't taken them or even really paid attention to them in my diet. I ate little of the fatty fish famous for omega-3 fats such as salmon, herring and sardines. But at that point I was desperate.

So I bought some omega-3 supplements, with some moderate dose of EPA and DHA and took some.

Now, I am not making this up. A few hours later I was sitting on the sofa perhaps watching TV, when suddenly my eyes started *gushing* tears. They were running down my cheeks. As if a tap had been turned on and would not turn off. It was bizarre. And I realized this could be an effect of the omega-3 fats. According to the American Academy of Ophthalmology, omega-3 fatty acids improve function of the meibomian glands, which are involved with tear production. My eyes had finally gotten enough of a key nutrient to begin making tears again.

While it took awhile longer to feel like my dry eye was under good control, I was a believer for life. I've been taking omega-3 supplements since then, for almost 15 years at this point. I have no interest in experiencing that again.

Dry eye is annoying, distressing and has a negative impact on quality of life. It's more common in older women, and living in a dry climate makes it worse. Eye doctors are aware of the omega-3 connection, and many now prescribe high-dose omega-3 supplements for patients with dry eye. If you have this problem, hopefully your eye doctor is knowledgeable about omega-3 and can make recommendations depending on the severity of your situation.

Age-Related Macular Degeneration (AMD)

The macula is a small and highly pigmented oval spot near the center of the retina. The yellow pigments are the carotenoids zeaxanthin and lutein, which act as a sort of natural sunblock, absorbing blue-ultraviolet light waves. As they block light waves, they are degraded, so your eyes need a constant source of replacement pigments.

Age-Related Macular Degeneration (AMD) develops over time as the macula is degrades. About ¼ of adults over age 65 have some macular degeneration, and According to the American Academy of Ophthalmology, it's the leading cause of blindness. Smoking, obesity and high saturated fat diets are linked to increased risk for AMD. People with high intakes of lutein and zeaxanthin from food have lower risk.

There is no official recommended daily intake for lutein and zeaxanthin. Diet intake data suggests that just 6 mg of lutein+zeaxanthin is linked to lower risk for AMD, but average intake in the US is more like 2-4 mg/day. Poor intake of vegetables and certain other foods would explain that number. Examples of foods with high levels of these two carotenes include:

½ cup cooked frozen spinach	15 mg
½ cup cooked kale	25 mg
1 cup cooked green peas	4 mg
1 cup cooked summer squash	4 mg
1 cup raw spinach	3.5 mg
1 cup cooked Brussels sprouts	2.4 mg
1 cup cooked broccoli	2 mg

Other foods with significant content include corn (and cornmeal), all other greens, asparagus, pumpkin, leeks, lettuce, oranges, tomatoes, egg (yolk), green beans, sweet and chili peppers and of course, carrots. So it's not hard to have a significant intake of these two important carotenes if you eat a variety of vegetables everyday.

Can a high intake of these two carotenes prevent AMD? At the moment we do not have good data to answer this question one way or another. Studies of AMD, such as the long term Age-Related Eye Diseases Study (AREDS) from the National Eye Institute focus on people who already have existing AMD. Subjects took high dose supplements and progression of AMD was measured. A well-designed study on prevention would take years. Subjects' intake from food would need to be assessed, along with blood levels of the nutrients in question. The AREDS did not assess blood levels of lutein and zeaxanthin, which is a major study design drawback in my opinion.

But why wait for a study? It's not hard to consume significant amounts of these two pigments from foods. The foods listed above have particularly high content of lutein and zeaxanthin, but many more vegetables and fruits have at least some. Add it all up for a day and you can easily consume the minimal 6 mg, and certainly more if you eat leafy dark greens on a regular basis.

Cataracts

According to the National Eye Institute, more than half of us will have developed a cataract by age 80. Cataracts progress over years, as proteins in the eye lens are damaged, causing cloudiness. In addition to age, risk factors include family history, smoking, diabetes and unprotected exposure to ultraviolet sunlight. Diet has not been investigated extensively as a risk factor, although experts believe that certain antioxidants, such as vitamins C and E, can protect the lenses from damage.

Long term diet intake studies link higher intakes of vitamin C to lower rates of cataracts. However, more isn't necessarily better. Moderate doses (60-250 mg per day) may have a long term benefit, but long-term mega-doses (1000 mg/day) have been associated with higher incidence of cataracts.

Other studies suggest that long term use of supplements that include C and E reduce risk. Lutein and zeaxanthin intake are also linked to lower cataract risk. But as with AMD, there are no studies examining whether long term (or life-long) high intake of any of these nutrients actually prevents cataracts.

Despite the lack of proof, there's no reason not to play it smart when it comes to food choices. Vitamin C is abundant in fruits and vegetables, many of which are also good sources of lutein and zeaxanthin. Vitamin E is concentrated in oils, nuts and nut butters. Most multiple vitamins have both of these nutrients in moderate doses.

Glaucoma

A check up visit to the eye doctor invariably includes tests for glaucoma. This serious eye disease results from damage to the optic nerve, caused by elevated pressure in the eye (Intra Ocular Pressure, or IOP).

Of all the serious eye diseases of aging, glaucoma is the least researched in terms of nutrition risk factors. There is a strong association with family history (genetics), but genetic factors don't account for all known risk.

Of course, there is interest in possible environmental risk factors. IOP can be raised, if only temporarily, by things like playing a wind instrument, doing certain head-down yoga postures or wearing a necktie. In most cases, IOP quickly returns to normal after the activity is complete or the necktie is loosened, so don't imagine that yoga or ties cause glaucoma.

A nutrition connection is even less apparent. Diet intake studies haven't shown a link between antioxidant intake or omega-3 intake and glaucoma. The AREDS initially excluded subjects with existing glaucoma. After 5 years on the study supplement (Vitamins C and E, zinc and lutein/zeaxanthin), IOP was not different between placebo and supplement groups. Which isn't to say there aren't other nutrients involved with glaucoma risk. Just that these particular nutrients do not appear to impact IOP or glaucoma risk.

Retinal Health

The retina lines the back of the eye. It's composed of 3 layers of rods and cones, which are light-sensitive. When light strikes the retina, the rods and cones convert the light to nerve impulses, which are sent to the optic nerve to facilitate visual images. This process depends on various molecular forms of vitamin A.

The retina has the highest concentration of polyunsaturated fatty acids, especially DHA, of any body tissue. It's subjected to considerable oxidative stress, so nutrition could impact retinal integrity.

The retina is subject to many disease processes. Diabetic retinopathy is a well-known side effect of diabetes, although the causes are not well understood. Retinal detachment or retinal tears become more common with age, although the reasons for this aren't clear. Some retinal diseases have known nutrition connections, such as retinitis pigmentosa. Vitamin A and DHA are sometimes used in treatment for some forms of this disease.

Despite the fact that the retina is very dependent on certain key nutrients, there isn't a lot of research on the relationship between retinal function or integrity and nutrition. The AREDS focused on the macula, which is a small specialized part of the retina. The best you can do is to maintain a high intake of nutrients that are generally good for eye health, including adequate – but not excessive – vitamin A, preferably from vegetables and fruits.

Eye Supplements

When research links medical conditions to nutrients, supplement manufacturers are not far behind. Eye health is one example. Multiple vitamin formulas for seniors are now sprinkled with a variety of carotenes and other eye-related nutrients like omega-3 fats, so the label can claim "supports eye health!"

The label of one brand name multivitamin brags about the

lutein content of 250 micrograms. Remember, the AREDS recommends 6 mg (or 6000 micrograms) of a lutein/zeaxanthin combination per day. 250 mcg is a trivial amount; you can get vastly more from a half cup of cooked spinach. When shopping for supplements, beware of Health Halo claims that aren't backed up by meaningful nutrient doses.

There is one specific eye health supplement based on the formula that showed the most benefit in the AREDS2. It's recommended by the American Academy of Ophthalmology as an intervention for AMD, although it is not promoted as a cure. This is a high dose formula of a limited number of nutrients:

- 500 mg vitamin C
- 400 IU vitamin E
- 80 mg zinc
- 10 mg lutein
- 2 mg zeaxanthin
- 2 mg copper (to counteract high dose zinc)

Copper is added to balance the effects of the high dose of zinc, not because copper has any particular benefit for eye health. Beta carotene, used in the original study, was replaced by lutein and zeaxanthin in the second part of the study. Because those were found to have a more beneficial effect, the final supplement formula contains those carotenes.

The formula is available from a number of supplement manufacturers, but it's specifically indicated for AMD, not for general eye health, because of the high doses. If you are developing AMD, your eye doctor may recommend this supplement. Check the nutrition facts panel before buying. Some manufacturers add other nutrients to the formula, or change the doses of the key nutrients. In some cases this might not be a problem, since some of them (ex: zinc) are very high. To avoid confusion, ask your doctor for a specific brand recommendation.

Other supplement manufacturers may create eye health formulas with specific nutrients for general eye health, not specifically for AMD. There is no evidence at the moment that megadoses of any nutrients are necessary to maintain eye health. There's also no evidence that some other unique nutrient formula has any particular benefit for eye health. You can get all of the key nutrients from a general purpose multiple vitamin/mineral.

While some multiples may include small amounts of omega-3 fatty acids, one pill cannot contain a meaningful dose. Adding a separate omega-3 supplement, or adding high omega-3 foods to your diet is the most effective way to boost intake.

Do you even need to take a special eye health supplement? Not if you:

- Eat a plant-based diet full of vegetables that are good sources of all those important carotenes
- Get adequate omega-3 fats from food and/or a supplement
- Take an all-purpose senior formula multiple vitamin/mineral

Take Away

We've come a long way from the idea that all you need is carrots. In fact, it turns out carrots aren't that special for eyes after all, compared to vegetables high in other carotenoids. Since we do know that those are important, one of the best pieces of advice for eye health is to eat a variety of vegetables and fruit. There it no downside to that. Those foods are loaded with plenty of other nutrients, plus fiber. Unless you have active eye disease that requires medical intervention, and your eye doctor has recommended some specific supplement as part of treatment, diet should be your main strategy for healthy eyes.

Even if you don't have active eye disease, you might be thinking, why not add a vision supplement, just for insurance? There is no standard vision formula. Every manufacturer invents their own, hopefully with input from actual research results. Most have some amount of lutein and perhaps zeaxanthin. I wouldn't take one that didn't include both, and in meaningful amounts. Remember that the suggested lutein intake is 6 mg/day, although the AREDS2 formula contains 10 mg. Amounts above that may or may not have any additional benefit. Just beware of lutein or zeaxanthin doses listed as *micro*grams to make the amount look impressive. 300 micrograms might sound good, but it's a mere 0.3 mg.

What about omega-3. Clearly omega-3 fatty acids, particularly DHA, play an important role in eye health, from structure to function to tear formation. If canola oil, flax and walnuts are part of your daily diet, you'll be consuming omega-3 as alpha-linolenic acid. This molecule must be metabolized to DHA before it helps your eyes; the conversion rate in humans is low, maybe 5-15%. If you're a fan of high omega-3 fish like salmon or sardines, and you consistently eat those a couple of times a week, you're probably consuming sufficient omega-3 as DHA and EPA. But if none of these foods are on your radar screen, you might consider a supplement. Chapter 12 has more information about choosing omega-3 supplements. Vision supplements are discussed in Chapter 13.

At the moment, we don't have enough information to say that boosting your intake of eye nutrients will reverse existing eye diseases. If you have a specific problem, you need input from an eye doctor. Nutrition should be part of any plan, but is not the whole plan.

11 BRAIN HEALTH

Where are my keys?

What's that person's name?

What did I go to the basement for? (Could the basement stairwell be shooting mind-eraser rays?)

We all know about this forgetfulness stuff, sometimes referred to as age-related cognitive decline. We can laugh at it or we can worry that it's a sign of something worse. It's a safe bet that everyone would prefer to prevent the progression of garden-variety forgetfulness to full-blown dementia.

Dementia is a degenerative syndrome that affects language skills, memory, emotions, attentiveness and problem solving. We tend to equate dementia with Alzheimer's disease, but in fact there are many causes for dementia. Alzheimer's is just one. Stroke, neurodegenerative disorders, certain vitamin deficiencies, alcoholism and traumatic brain injury, such as from concussions, can predispose a person to dementia.

So we can all agree we'd rather avoid dementia, whatever the cause. Can it be prevented with diet and lifestyle changes? Can it be reversed once it's started? These are the $64 questions. Certainly prevention would be preferable to years of deteriorating quality of life and expensive specialized medical care.

Unfortunately research dollars are focused on finding drugs that reverse or stabilize people with dementia. That's where the money is. Researching the nutrition connection to age-related dementia in a manner that yields meaningful and actionable results would probably be prohibitively complicated and expensive. You'd have to sign up thousands of people at a young age and follow them into old age, monitoring everything from diet to exercise to weight, genetics and medical conditions. Everything about their environment would have to be documented, from water supply to work to family structure to transportation to geographical location.

That's not going to happen. At the moment, research on nutrition-related factors sounds like so much 'locking-the-barn-door-after-the-horse-has-been-stolen'. A group of elderly people is recruited, sometimes already showing signs of mild cognitive impairment. Some nutrition supplement is given or diet records are collected; progression of cognitive impairment or mood is assessed with standard tests and/or brain scans. Results are compared to nutrient intake. At best the conclusion might be that some nutrient or type of diet slows progression of impairment.

One thing we can safely assume is that the factors that predispose someone to cognitive impairment or dementia in later life start years earlier. So prevention probably needs to start at a young age. Does that mean diet and nutrition are pointless for older adults. I personally and professionally do *not* believe that. Alzheimer's disease is devastating, and I certainly don't want to lead people on with false promises of cures. But I do think some of what we refer to as dementia or cognitive impairment can be ameliorated by diet and lifestyle.

Maybe that's the best we can hope for at the moment: slower progression and less severe impairment. The brain is vastly complicated, but that doesn't mean at some point in the future we'll be able to intervene to keep older adults sharp, so they remember why they went to the basement.

Brain Structure

Our brains are built with nutrients, starting in the womb. All nutrients are important for this process, but some are especially important at the different stages of fetal brain development. Deficiencies can adversely impact brain structure, neuron organization and brain chemistry. Protein, zinc, iron, copper, iodine, folate, vitamin A, choline, selenium and omega-3 fats are especially important. Other substances, such as certain antioxidants, can also impact brain function in beneficial ways.

The adult human brain weighs about 3 pounds and is 60% fat. Omega-3 fatty acids – particularly DHA -- are critically important, because of their unique molecular shape. They are part of cell membrane structure and are the building blocks for several neurotransmitters and immune modulators.

What happens if you don't consume sufficient omega-3 fats to support brain structure and function? Rodent studies show that other fats are substituted in brain tissue, but omega-6 polyunsaturated fats, saturated fats and trans fats have very different molecular shapes and behavior then omega-3 fats. Cell membranes "designed" to utilize the biochemical characteristics of omega-3 fatty acids might not work so well when saturated or trans fats are substituted in. It's like designing a wall to be build with rectangular bricks, but the supplier only delivers square bricks. You can piece something together, but it's not done according to the original design. The integrity of the wall can be compromised.

Despite that very high fat content, fat is not the preferred fuel for brain cells. That is glucose. The brain uses about 70% of your available glucose every day, even though it represents only about 2% of your body weight. The need for a constant supply of glucose can explain why you get mentally fatigued or cranky when you're really hungry. Symptoms of hypoglycemia -- abnormally low blood sugar – include anxiety, confusion and irritability, which progress as the brain is deprived of fuel.

The nutritional building blocks that make brain cells work must be replenished throughout life. It's not unreasonable to conclude that decades of poor diet would adversely impact brain function.

Mood, Depression and Anxiety

We've all experienced depression or anxiety from time to time. But major depressive disorder is more than just a situational bad mood. It's a debilitating endless bad mood that severely impacts quality of life. The WHO estimates that the global disease burden of depression will be second only to heart disease by 2020. It affects women twice as often as men, and the personal, social and economic consequences are considerable.

According to the CDC's Healthy Aging Program:

"Depression is not a normal part of growing older... [It is] a true and treatable medical condition, not a normal part of aging. However older adults are at an increased risk for experiencing depression"

The CDC has a long list of potential signs of depression, including:

- Sadness and anxiety that last for weeks
- Feelings of hopelessness, guilt, pessimism and helplessness
- Irritability, fatigue, decreased energy
- Difficulty concentrating
- Aches, pains, cramps and digestive problems that do not improve with treatment
- Sleep disturbances and insomnia

The brain is enormously complicated. There are different regions that control different sets of functions, from breathing and heart beat to sight to language and thinking. There are trillions of nerve cell connections. The cells in each region certainly have structural and metabolic similarities, but they also have key differences. It's also not clear that any one region is responsible for depression. Dysfunction in one or more regions could trigger symptoms we describe as depression.

Because of this extreme complexity, it's unlikely that optimal nutrition is the universal cure for major depression. But there is a growing body of evidence that diet and certain nutrients do affect chronic mood and anxiety disorders. It seems like common sense, since nutrients are the building blocks of brain structure and brain chemistry.

One meta analysis of the combined data from 21 studies found that a so-called "healthy" diet pattern – high in fruits, vegetables, fish and whole grains -- was associated with less depression. However a "Western" diet pattern – high fat, high sugar, processed foods – was *not* significantly linked to *more* depression.

To add further confusion, some of the studies that were reviewed produced unexpected results:

- Healthy Japanese diet linked to higher risk for depression
- Meat, poultry and dairy foods not linked to depression
- High intake of fruits and vegetables linked to more depression
- Processed meat decreased risk for depression in women
- High intake of starchy foods linked to more depression symptoms

That last one probably rings a bell for some people. It's believed that people self-medicate with high simple carb starchy/sweet foods when in an anxious/depressed mood. And there's a biochemical explanation for that. Carbohydrates stimulate production of serotonin, a mood enhancing brain chemical. The beneficial effect might be fleeting, not to mention counter-productive, if it leads to excess calories or generally poor diet. But many people have experienced this situation.

The bigger unknown for this type of study is causation. Do "healthy" diets reduce depression? Or are happier people more likely to be eating that healthier diet, as well as engaging in other healthier behaviors like exercise or social interactions? Are depressed anxious people more likely to pick processed foods high in sugar, starch or fat? Or does that type of diet *cause* depression? This study does not answer that question.

Other studies have linked long-term adherence to a Mediterranean diet with less risk for major depression. One key feature of this type of diet is the high intake of monounsaturated fats from olive oil. In fact, rodent studies show that a high intake of monounsaturated fat improves brain insulin resistance, dopamine signaling and cell membrane integrity. Depression-like behaviors are reduced. And yes, researchers have ways to measure depression-like behavior in mice without calling in a mouse psychologist.

The Mediterranean diet link makes sense for another reason: gut microbes. As noted in the chapter about gut microbes (Chapter 9), the gut and brain communicate by way of the gut-brain axis. Rodent and human studies show that certain gut microbe populations can predispose to depression or anxiety-like behaviors. A plant-based Mediterranean-style diet, high encourages a population of beneficial gut microbes.

Omega-3 fats are another research focus, because of their important role in brain function. Again, much of the data is from mouse studies, and results do suggest a link between depression and poor omega-3 status. In humans, there is similar evidence. Studies that compare blood levels of omega-3 fats to depression incidence tend to show that the higher the levels of omega-3 fatty acids in blood, the lower the risk for depression. Other studies show that subjects with depression tend to have lower levels of omega-3 in their blood.

Diet surveys back up these findings, although not always. Studies that rely on peoples' ability to provide accurate reports of long-term food intake don't always give meaningful information. Analysis of brain tissue fatty acids would be even more useful, but this would not be feasible for living human subjects. However, there have been post-mortem studies of brain tissue composition that compared the brains of people with depressive disorders to people without such diagnoses. Again, the depressed subjects had lower omega-3 in brain tissue.

In another interesting twist, researchers are looking at the possibility that omega-3 fats may improve depression treatment by improving response to anti-depressant medications, resulting in more effective outcomes.

Are omega-3 fats a cure for depression? It would be

irresponsible to make that claim. Yes the evidence points to a connection. Given the importance of omega-3 fatty acids to brain integrity, it just makes sense that poor omega-3 status would have an adverse impact on brain function, probably in multiple ways. The problem is, we don't have a good definition for optimal, let alone poor, omega-3 status. There is no consensus on the definition of a recommended intake. There is no consensus on optimal blood levels, let alone what exactly to measure in blood.

Major depressive disorder is multi-factorial. Genetics and environment certain play a role. Many medical conditions, such as hypothyroid, predispose to depression. Grief, loss and other serious or not-so-serious life disruptions can push you into bouts of depression, anxiety or both. Poor nutritional status may make you more susceptible or impede treatment and recovery. Good nutritional status may help you cope by making you more resilient.

What should you do?

If you are not suffering from major depressive disorder or debilitating anxiety, have never experienced these and have no family history, then you may be more resilient to the emotional impact of adverse life events. Perhaps you already have a wonderful diet. Or perhaps you have good genes. If you have been diagnosed, and treatment is going well, eating a better diet and improving omega-3 intake won't hurt. If you are living with significant depression, diagnosed by a physician, and treatment is not providing enough improvement, diet and nutrition should be part of your long term strategy.

If you're considering adding omega-3 supplements, read through the omega-3 section in Chapter 12. Remember, nutrients, such as omega-3 fatty acids, are not drugs. They do not produce dramatic overnight results, as an antibiotic or steroid might. So dosing yourself with omega-3 supplements isn't going to eliminate your depression in a day or two.

How much? As I noted, health experts can't even agree on an optimal intake for healthy people, so there is no standard recommendation for medical conditions like major depressive disorder.   Studies can provide some guidance.   In general, studies on humans show that a 1 to 2 grams supplement of omega-3 daily was sufficient to improve symptoms.   If you don't like the idea of supplements, eating high omega-3 fish, such as salmon, at least twice a week is a good plan.   Herring, mackerel and sardines are also good omega-3 sources; tuna less so.

Don't rely on omega-3 fatty acids alone.   The impact of the whole diet can't be discounted, especially considering the beneficial effects of gut microbes.   A plant-centric diet encourages those beneficial microbes.

Cognition

Cognition -- thinking, memory, learning, language -- takes place in the brain, so it makes sense that nutrition could affect mental sharpness as much as depression.   Mental acuity declines with age.   Risk for dementia goes up.   The possibility of preventing or reversing any degree of mental impairment with nutrition or food is very compelling.

Genetics, environment, smoking, diseases, medical treatments and other factors all impact brain function and cognitive integrity.   Scientific studies investigating the link between nutrition and cognition provide some hints about benefits, but so far no solid evidence for cause-and-effect prevention or cures.

Of course, lack of evidence doesn't bother some people. There are plenty of cognition-boosting claims for various diets, foods, herbs, nutrients, antioxidants and amino acids. Many of the claims are based on anecdotal testimonials or pure speculation. But desperate people dealing with the devastating effects of dementia can't always distinguish between evidence and marketing.

Here's a list of foods, nutrients and medical conditions currently on the cognition-nutrition radar screen:

1. **Lutein and zeaxanthin**: these antioxidants were discussed in the chapter on eye health (Chapter 10). They're important for vision, and research shows

that they also accumulate in brain tissue. Low levels are associated with cognitive impairment. A lutein supplementation study of older women showed improvements in memory, learning and verbal fluency.

2. **Vitamin D**: insufficient blood levels are associated with increased risk for developing dementia and Alzheimer's disease. Does low vitamin D increase dementia risk? Perhaps. Or perhaps low vitamin D is a marker for a diet and lifestyle that contributes to cognitive impairment. But it's not a bad idea to make sure your vitamin D is at a healthy level. And of course, excessive vitamin D will not improve brain function.

3. **Vitamin B12**: deficiency is a known risk factor for dementia, poor memory, confusion and depression. Again, excessive intake is not helpful. Having adequate B12 in blood is sufficient. One risk factor common for older adults: use of proton pump inhibitors or H2 receptor antagonist medications for ulcers or other stomach problems inhibits B12 absorption. If you are on these medications you should have your B12 checked.

4. **Obesity**: while obesity is linked to many chronic diseases, obesity itself, from middle age on, was linked to an acceleration of the loss of white matter in the brain normally associated with aging. Is this caused by the obesity itself, or the lifestyle that contributes to obesity? This question has not been answered.

5. **Omega-3 fatty acids**: Given the critical role of omega-3s in brain function, it's no surprise that intake is linked to mental acuity in older adults. Higher omega-3 intake is associated with better cognitive function in many studies, but not all. Study design may account for conflicting results. Short-term studies done on elderly people with existing cognitive impairment or outright dementia are not

likely to provide much in the way of meaningful results. By the time the disease has advanced, brain structure and function have been severely disrupted and the brain is subjected to adverse effects of inflammation. Expecting any one nutrient to reverse this situation is unrealistic.

In general, studies that compare blood levels of omega-3 fatty acids to cognition in healthy older adults link higher levels to better overall performance on cognitive tests and lower risk for developing Alzheimer's disease. There's also evidence that supplementation of omega-3/DHA along with other nutrients, such as certain B vitamins, produces better results than supplementing just omega-3.

The consensus of experts is that omega-3 fatty acids are important for brain integrity throughout life. Maintaining an adequate intake during adulthood is the best plan for supporting cognition in later years, although healthy older adults can benefit from increased intake even in later years.

Cognition boosting claims for many other nutrients, herbs and food components are proliferating. Here are some examples:

Choline: Because this vitamin-like nutrient is important for neuronal membrane function and neurotransmitter signaling, many studies have investigated the relationship between choline and cognitive decline. So far, there is no clear evidence that choline provides any particular benefit. Of course, getting sufficient choline remains important for health. The recommended daily intake for adult women is 425 mg. It's especially abundant in eggs, liver and wheat germ. Meats and fish are also decent sources.

B Vitamins in general: While it's important to get sufficient B-vitamins, there's no evidence that excess doses improve cognitive ability. Some diseases do interfere with some B vitamins, which can lead to brain effects, along with many other problems. For example, alcoholism is famous for depleting B1, which can severely impair brain function.

Alzheimer's disease patients frequently are thiamin-deficient because of poor diets and malabsorption. However, studies using supplemental B1 have not resulted in improvement of symptoms.

Lithium: This mineral is not a nutrient. It is used as a drug to treat bipolar disease. Because the drug form can impact brain function, it's been packaged up as an over-the-counter supplement, at much lower doses and in different chemical forms from the prescription drug. However, evidence that it has any impact on cognitive impairment or dementia is lacking.

Coconut oil: One theory about Alzheimer's disease claims that the problem is all about energy supply for brain cells. Glucose metabolism is disrupted, so if you can supply an alternative energy source, all will be well. Ketones, a by-product of fat metabolism, can be used for energy. The fats in coconut oil can be converted to ketones, so coconut oil proponents leap to the conclusion that therefore coconut oil helps Alzheimer's disease. According to the Alzheimer's Association (ALZ.org), there are no clinical studies confirming any benefit from coconut oil. Searching the PubMed database of clinical research returns no results for clinical studies of "coconut and Alzheimer's disease". Nevertheless there are plenty of products, websites, books and assorted anecdotes claiming that coconut oil helps Alzheimer's, usually attached to a sales pitch for a coconut oil product. Draw your own conclusions.

Ketogenic Diet: this diet ties in to the claims for coconut oil, namely that ketones are a good energy source for brain cells. The ketogenic diet has been around for decades as a therapy for seizures. For reasons not entirely clear, this extremely high fat diet, which leads to metabolic ketosis, suppresses seizures. It's still used for children who have intractable seizures. It's not an easy diet to follow. People with Alzheimer's or other dementias can have seizures, so the theory grew that a ketogenic diet should be helpful.

In fact some research suggests that for mild to moderate cases of Alzheimer's disease, ketogenic diets can provide some modest benefit for cognitive function. Key word: modest.

Other keyword: mild-to-moderate cases. Undoubtedly there will be more research on this. Ketogenic diets may be useful as part of overall therapy, not as a cure.

The biggest problem is the diet itself, which is 70% fat. It's extremely monotonous and unpalatable, and would require careful daily attention to cooking and meals. Another side effect is weight loss. In fact ketogenic diets are also promoted for weight loss. But people with dementia frequently have a difficult time maintaining weight; they don't need a weight loss diet.

Plenty of other substances are promoted to enhance cognitive function or treat dementia. The list seems to grow weekly. At the moment there is little-to-no evidence for any benefit; in many cases studies show zero benefit:

- Vitamin E
- Ginko
- Bee pollen
- Niacin
- A derivative of colostrum
- Lemon balm
- Melatonin
- Rosemary
- Ginseng
- Vinpocetine
- Creatine
- Whey protein
- Green tea

The list could go on and on. Suffice it to say that if any of these ever show remarkable benefits for people with dementia, or for people experiencing age-related cognitive impairment, it will be big news. You won't hear anything like "well 10 people seemed to benefit, but another 25 people had no benefit".

Your Brain On Food

It's great to know there is so much evidence for foods and nutrients that do help your brain. Now what do you do with that information?

Depression and age-related cognitive decline are complex degenerative processes with many contributing factors, including genetics, medications, lifestyle, environment, substance abuse, disease states and nutrition.

Of all the possible nutrition-related factors, some stand out to me as especially important in terms of brain health and as related to the diet and nutrition issues of aging. In my professional opinion, these are:

1. Overall diet
2. Omega-3 fatty acids
3. B12
4. Gut microbiome
5. Everything else.

It's more of a Big Picture concept. Brain function depends on many nutrients, all present at optimal levels. Cognitive impairment and depression are not caused by a lack of ginseng or ketones or coconut. Cognitive decline is not going to be fixed by any one nutrient or food.

The nutrition-cognition research consistently points to a link between a plant-based Mediterranean style diet and better mental acuity. There are probably many reasons for this. Thanks to the plant foods, this diet is loaded with nutrients, antioxidants, carotenes like lutein, fiber and carbohydrates that encourage a healthy gut microbe population and healthy fats. Traditional Mediterranean style diets have significant amounts of fish, which means significant omega-3 fats. Dairy, especially fermented foods like yogurt, along with eggs provide high quality protein, additional vitamins, including B12, and minerals.

If you're not into eating much fish, supplementing with omega-3 is an option. If you don't eat much meat or dairy, B12 can definitely be a problem. This is especially true of you take medications that interfere with B12 absorption, in which case a supplement may be advisable. Having your B12 status checked with blood analysis will determine if supplementation is necessary.

Encouraging beneficial gut bacteria depends completely on food choices. You can take a probiotic supplement hoping that it helps, but if you don't eat the foods to encourage those microbes, a supplement isn't going to do much. And that means plant foods. So we get right back to a plant-based diet. You'll find more information in the final chapter.

Finally...

After writing down all this carefully worded information about brain health and nutrition, I want to get real. This is important stuff. The research is relatively recent. We are one of the first generations that can take advantage of this information and put it to good use, for our own health and well-being. The research in ongoing. More information will become clearer in the future. It's likely that the outlines of a brain health diet and lifestyle will evolve. Such a diet might not preserve every neuron and synapse, but as long as we can live our lives with a high level of mental and physical vitality, who cares if sometimes we forget why we're in the basement?

12 SUPPLEMENTS – SINGLE NUTRIENTS

"Nutrition, line 1. Nutrition, line 1"
Nothing makes me crazier than hearing that over the P.A. system in a grocery store. I'm surrounded by food, much of it lovely, loaded with nutrients. But where is the "nutrition" in this store? It's in the pill section. What's the purpose of all the food then? Entertainment? Guilty pleasure?

Until very recently in human history, nutrition meant food and nothing but food. Hippocrates famously said "Let food be thy medicine." People had a vague idea that there were things in some foods that helped in specific ways. The realization that scurvy on long ocean voyages could be prevented by limes is one example, leading to the nickname "Limeys" for British sailors. But nutrients weren't really identified and isolated as unique molecules until the 20th century. In the mid-20th century, industrial scale manufacture of vitamins took off, and supplements became commonplace after WWII.

Nobel laureate Linus Pauling, a chemist by training, branched off into nutritional biochemistry, and became fascinated by vitamin C. He believed large doses of vitamin C would prevent or cure just about every disease known to man, from the common cold to cancer. The era of vitamin supplements escalated at that point. People were sold on the idea that a nice natural-sounding vitamin would fix all their problems. Despite years of research, evidence for vitamin C's magical powers was never established. But that doesn't bother plenty of people; even today if you go to a vitamin or "health food" store, you'll likely find an entire aisle devoted to vitamin C alone.

Until the mid-20th century, humans survived for millions of years without supplements. Now all known nutrients can be bought in a pill. You can get combinations of nutrients. You can buy herbal "supplements", although there is no daily herb requirement. Why are we so obsessed with taking pills? I don't know the answer; I'm not sure anyone does. Buying over-the-counter natural-sounding pills to hopefully make yourself healthier is a very attractive idea. Sort of like do-it-yourself medicine.

Usage data shows that almost half of US adults use supplements. Sixty-four percent of adults over age 62 report supplement use. We spend almost $40 billion a year on supplements. Keep in mind, those are not covered by insurance. Those are out-of-pocket expenses, yet people are willing to spend the money.

While supplements may or may not do you any good, usually they are not dangerous. The FDA regulates supplements only to the extent that they:

1. Contain what the label says they contain
2. Do not cause harm or illness

The FDA does not care if a supplement actually provides a health benefit. There are no laws to that effect. The label cannot suggest a supplement cures or prevents any disease. So you see statements like "supports bone health" or "supports immune function". Or no statement at all. Some multiples now contain a dusting of probiotics or antioxidants. Those are health halo words, so just seeing "Contains Probiotics!" on the label will be enough for many consumers to conclude that a particular multiple is a healthier choice.

Why take a supplement?

When I surveyed women about topics for this book, supplements was the topic picked by almost everyone. I thought that was really interesting, but I realized I forgot to ask "why?" Because people are taking supplements and want some clarification about them? Because people *aren't* taking them, and think maybe they should? Or aren't taking them and are looking for validation about their choice?

In fact I can address all those possibilities. There are reasons for and against supplements, depending on your health and your diet. You might think you should take supplements because you've heard that supplement users are healthier. But of course, supplement users may have generally healthier lifestyles. It's not the supplements making people healthy; rather it's the interest in health that leads to purchase supplements. On the other hand, some research shows that supplement users have higher circulating levels of nutrients than non-users. Not surprising; the significant question is this: are you *healthier* because you have higher levels of some nutrients? That's not necessarily a given.

There is one rather significant rationale for taking certain supplements as we age. Our metabolism slows down. We need fewer calories, and therefore less food each day. But we do *not* require lower doses of most nutrients. So you'd have to eat an increasingly healthier more nutrient-dense, junk-free diet as the years go on. If you're going to get all your vitamins and minerals from food, there would be less and less, or zero, room for nutrient-poor foods. Are you willing to be that vigilant about your daily food choices?

Some other common effects of aging can also impact nutrient requirements:

1. Body composition changes – less muscle mass, more fat mass
2. Changes in taste
3. Changes in physiological function, including decreased vitamin absorption
4. Changes in immune function
5. Decreased functionality of some organs

I'm not advocating that everyone take supplements. I'm not suggesting that supplements are pointless. I can give you reasons for and against certain ones, so you can make your own decision. You might conclude something makes sense for you; you might conclude that something you're taking now doesn't make much sense. Hopefully you'll be a more informed consumer when you're shopping the supplement aisle.

This chapter is about supplements that could be useful for older women. I outline the reasons for them and give you some information about different forms and doses you are likely to find at the store. I take some of these myself, although not necessarily every day. Remember, they're *supplements*. They just supposed to supplement your intake from food, not replace it.

Label Terminology

When buying supplements, there are a few terms you should be familiar with:

RDA: Recommended dietary allowance is the amount of a nutrient that will meet the daily requirement of 97.5% of the population of a particular age/gender group.

DRI: Dietary reference intakes are the whole set of nutrient values, intended to define recommended nutrient intakes that fit the needs of healthy people.

% DV: This is typically how supplement and Nutrition Facts labels describe the dose of each nutrient included. DV refers to Daily Value, which is a *very* general one-size-fits all dose for someone eating 2000 calories/day. Most women, especially older women, eat fewer calories than that. So if you eat about 1500 calories/day, you might be fine with 75% of the DV for those nutrients. Even more confusing, the DV does not always correspond to the RDA for a person in a specific age group, although the numbers aren't typically that different. For example, the DV for calcium is 1000 mg, but the RDA for an older women is 1200 mg. The DV for vitamin D is 400 IU, but for older adults it's now 600 IU. So %DV on a supplement label is useful in a limited way to assess how the amount of a nutrient in a food or supplement compares to a daily recommendation.

AI: Adequate Intake is an estimated dose that's expected to cover everyone's needs for that nutrient. Nutrients with no established RDA will have an AI instead. AI is used when there isn't sufficient information to establish an RDA for daily intake of a nutrient for a particular age/gender group. What's the AI based on? Sometimes it's based on the mean intakes of a population group.   For example, AI values are common for infant nutrient recommendations, as there is not much research done on infants (it would not be ethical). And AI values are more common for trace minerals, for which there is not much research on intake. Chromium and manganese are two examples.

International Units (IU), activity units and gram weights: Values for fat soluble vitamins – A, D and E – are given in a variety of measurement units. IU was the traditional unit of measurement, but Activity Units are used more widely now.   This is a way to compare the biological activity of different forms of each of these vitamins. For example, active vitamin A, retinol, is present in some foods. But vitamin A precursor molecules in plant foods – such as beta-carotene, alpha-carotene and beta-cryptoxanthin – have different structures which must first be converted to active vitamin A. Rather than expect everyone to sort out all the different forms, the vitamin A measurement is given in activity units, or Retinol Activity Equivalents (RAE). 1 microgram (μg) of retinol is one RAE.   12 micrograms of beta-carotene = 1 RAE, while 24 micrograms of alpha-carotene is 1 RAE. So beta-carotene is more potent than alpha-carotene. The same type of system applies to the different forms of vitamin D and vitamin E (tocopherols).

Here's a list of RDAs and AIs for most known nutrients for women in our age range (µg = micrograms):

Nutrient	Amount/day	Other info
Vitamin A	700 µg	Or 700 RAE
Vitamin C	75 mg	
Vitamin D	15-20 µg	600-800 IU
Vitamin E	15 mg	
Vitamin K	90 µg	AI
B1	1.1 mg	Thiamin
B2	1.1 mg	Riboflavin
Niacin	14 mg	
B6	1.5 mg	Pyridoxine
Folate	400 µg	
B12	2.4 µg	Cobalamin
Pantothenic Acid	5 mg	AI
Biotin	30 µg	AI
Choline	425 mg	AI
Calcium	1200 mg	
Chromium	20 µg	AI
Copper	900 µg	
Iodine	150 µg	
Iron	8 mg	
Magnesium	320 mg	
Manganese	1.8 mg	AI
Molybdenum	45 µg	
Phosphorus	700 mg	
Selenium	55 µg	
Zinc	8 mg	
Potassium	4700 mg	AI

1 gram = 1,000 mg = 1,000,000 µg ; 1 mg = 1000 µg

Vitamin A

Let's start with the one vitamin you might not need more of as you age. The term "vitamin A" actually refers to a group of fat-soluble molecules. Retinol, retinal and retinoic acid are the active forms of this vitamin; carotenoids, from vegetables and fruit, must be metabolized to active forms in the body, but only about 10% of known carotenoids can be transformed to vitamin A.

Active vitamin A is essential for numerous metabolic functions, such as eyesight, immune function and gene expression. It's found in animal-sourced foods such as liver, eggs, milk and cheese. It's also added to some fortified foods, such as ready-to-eat cereals, and is the form of vitamin A included in many multiples. Carotenoids are plentiful in orange and dark green vegetables (spinach, sweet potato, carrots, broccoli) and fruits (cantaloupe, apricots, mango).

Because it's fat soluble, excess vitamin A is not flushed out of the body. Active vitamin A is stored in the liver. Carotenoids are not automatically metabolized to active vitamin A; that depends on your need for vitamin A. Unused carotenoids can accumulate in tissues. In fact, the skin of people who consistently eat very large amounts of high carotenoid foods can take on an orange hue.

Having an orange skin tone might look unusual, but is not known to be unhealthy. Having excess vitamin A stored in your liver is unhealthy, and can lead to toxicity symptoms. Liver function declines with age, leaving older people more susceptible to toxicity.

The solution is pretty simple. Avoid supplements of active vitamin A: retinol, retinal and retinoic acid. Many supplements for seniors now use carotenoids instead, which are clearly listed on the supplement label. Even better: eat plenty of dark-colored vegetables and fruits, in a meal with some fat to enhance carotenoid absorption.

Vitamin A in supplements and fortified foods may be listed as International Units (IU) or Retinol Activity Equivalent (RAE), which is becoming the preferred descriptor. This levels the playing field, so to speak, among all the different forms of this vitamin. For example, 1 RAE equals 1 microgram of active vitamin A or 12 mcg of dietary beta carotene or 24 mcg of dietary beta cryptoxanthin. Meaning active vitamin A is more potent than the carotene in carrots.

Take Away: barring an unusual medical condition, you don't need separate vitamin A supplements. If you take a multiple, you're likely getting vitamin A. Check the ingredients list to verify that the carotenoid form is used. If you don't take a multiple, include plenty of dark orange/red or green vegetables and fruits in your diet. Just don't overdo those, or you might turn orange.

Calcium

There's been a lot of negative publicity about calcium supplements lately, linking them to heart disease risk. I'm not convinced the studies are all that conclusive, but I wouldn't recommend relying on pills for calcium everyday. The studies do suggest that getting most of your calcium from supplements alone – 1000 mg calcium/day from pills -- is a poor choice. Compared to a calcium pill, food has many other components, in particular other important nutrients related to bone health like protein and phosphorus.

The official recommendation for calcium for older women is 1200 mg/day. That's the equivalent of 4 servings of a high calcium dairy food, or four 300 mg pills. Given that other foods have some calcium, particularly some plant foods like greens or legumes, you will get calcium from everything you eat.

If you need to boost calcium you can do it by eating lots of high calcium foods daily. This means at least 3 servings of a dairy food such as milk, cheese, yogurt or kefir, or a calcium fortified beverage like soy milk. However, calcium fortified foods like soy milk are basically a beverage with a crushed up calcium pill added. Sort of like drinking a supplement.

There are several different forms of supplemental calcium, including:
- Calcium carbonate
- Calcium citrate
- Calcium malate
- Calcium lactate
- Calcium gluconate
- Oyster shell (carbonate form)
- Coral (carbonate form)
- Calcium hydroxyapatite (cow bone source)

There is also calcium derived from algae. There really isn't any evidence that one form is absorbed vastly better than another. There is evidence that, for older women, calcium citrate or malate may be better absorbed because we tend to lose stomach acidity as we age, and calcium carbonate relies more on an acidic environment for absorption. Calcium citrate is the preferred form to be used for older adults with intestinal problems such as inflammatory bowel disease.

These days calcium is typically combined with vitamin D. Some brands include other minerals like magnesium or zinc, or vitamin K2. All of these are linked to bone health. However, the amounts included in these combo preparations may or may not be significant. See Chapter 5 on bone health for more details on all the important nutrients for bones. If you take vitamin D separately, you need to add any amount from your calcium supplement to your daily total. See the vitamin D section below for more information.

One other thing to pay attention to: the amount of calcium *per tablet.* Frequently the label will say something like "1000 mg calcium per dose" followed by "suggested dose 3 tablets per day". In other words each tablet has 333 mg, not 1000 mg. Watch out for that. There's general agreement that your body can absorb up to 500 mg at any one time, so taking a handful of calcium pills all at once is not just a bad idea, it could be a waste.

I pay attention to my daily calcium intake for bone health, and I choose to use a combination of high calcium foods and 1 calcium citrate supplement – 300 mg -- a day. I go with 1-2 dairy foods, 1 pill and assume other foods make up the rest. I might get 900-1000 mg calcium a day, not 1200. I'm personally OK with that for myself.

Take Away: Relying only on pills to cover your calcium needs isn't a great idea. High calcium foods have other nutrients important for health, bone health in particular. If you do use a calcium supplement, citrate or malate are preferable for older women.

Vitamin D

Vitamin D is one of the most popular vitamin supplements of the 21st century (so far). Even doctors are on board; that's saying something. Vitamin D tests are now standard operating procedure for many medical practices, and with good reason. It turns out plenty of people have low levels, but don't know it. There aren't any obvious external signs for low vitamin D.

Technically vitamin D is more of a hormone than a true vitamin. In normal circumstances, vitamin D is made in skin cells when skin is exposed to sunshine. Specific ultraviolet wavelengths from the sun's rays cause metabolic changes in vitamin D precursor molecules in skin cells, changing the molecules to active vitamin D.

But circumstances aren't normal anymore. People spend very little time outside these days. We're either in a car or in a building. And when we do go outside, we slather up with sunscreen, which blocks the very rays that would be making vitamin D. Two other aspects of modern life also interfere with the sun-vitamin-D connection: air pollution that blocks the sun's rays and population shifts farther north, where sunshine is in short supply for months every year.

For older people, there is one more critical piece of the puzzle: even if you are outside in bright sunlight without sunscreen, older skin becomes less and less able to produce vitamin D. So for older adults, a vitamin D supplement may not just be a good idea; it may be essential.

The first step in deciding is a blood test. If your vitamin D level is in an acceptable range, whatever you're doing is working, no need for extra supplements. If not, then a supplement may be in order. But how much? With vitamin D, a big dose may not be the best choice.

There are two major problems:

1. No one can agree on what the optimal blood level range is.
2. There's no way to predict that, if you take XXXX mg of vitamin D your blood level will increase by XX ng/ml* after X months.

Which Blood Level?

Here are some examples of different institutions' ideas about what an adequate blood range for vitamin D is, given in nanograms per milliliter:

<u>National Institutes of Health:</u>
Deficient: less than 12 ng/ml
Generally Inadequate: 12-20
Adequate 20+
Potentially adverse effects with levels above 50.

<u>Vitamin D Council/Endocrine Society</u>
Severely deficient: less than 10 ng/ml
Deficient: 10-30
Adequate: 30-50 ng/ml
Greater than 100 ng/ml: potentially harmful, 150 is a toxic level.

What can we conclude in general?
- A level of less than 20 ng/ml is too low.
- If your level is in the 30's ng/ml you're probably adequate.
- Levels above 50 may be problematic, up to toxicity at 150 ng/ml

*Some labs give vitamin D results in nanomoles per liter (nmol/l); some use nanograms per milliliter (ng/ml). This can be confusing if you don't pay attention to the units being used. The nmol/l unit always comes out looking bigger. If you were thinking ng/ml, but looking at nmol/l, you might end up making a wrong conclusion about your vitamin D status. To convert, multiply the ng/ml value by 2.5 to get the nmol/l value. Or divide the nmol/l unit by 2.5 to get the ng/ml value.

Your blood test results will reflect whatever standard your lab uses. Some may flag levels below 30 as "low"; other labs may use 20 as the cut off point. Some labs may have a "normal" range of 20-100 ng/ml!

Research I've read recently about beneficial health effects of vitamin D indicate that levels between 30 and 40 ng/ml were linked to the best outcomes; levels above that didn't provide any additional benefit. So I'm inclined to be happy with my own level in the 30's, perhaps into the low 40's.

How Much?

The RDA for vitamin D for older adults is 600 International Units (IU) daily. IU refers to a unit of vitamin D activity, not to a weight. Sometimes the amounts are listed in micrograms. There are 4 IU per microgram.

Recommending a specific dose of vitamin D for everyone who reads this book is not appropriate, as everyone has a different situation and different health concerns. I do suggest that older women be tested. Then you know your baseline. Simply taking vitamin D supplements without knowing your blood level is a bad idea.

If you want to take a supplement to correct a low level, the first step after a blood test is some input from your physician. You can certainly purchase a wide range of doses. Some MDs prescribe big whopping once-a-month doses (say 100,000 IU) and re-test blood after 2-3 months. Some advise low dose daily supplements, of say 600-1000 IU. Find the cholecalciferol (D3) form and take any supplement with a meal that includes fats, as this is a fat soluble vitamin.

I average 1000-2000 IU per day, mostly from the amount in supplements. This maintains my blood level in an acceptable range. Dairy foods like milk and yogurt are fortified with D. If you spend lots of time outside in bright sunshine, you might still synthesize some in exposed skin.

Take Away: Get tested before starting a supplement regimen. You might not need extra D.

Vitamin K

We get vitamin K, the K1 phylloquinone form, from green leafy vegetables and some other fruits and vegetables. Another form, menaquinone, is found in certain fermented foods. The latest buzz is that this form, sometimes referred to as K2 or

MK-4 or MK-7, plays an important role in calcium metabolism, impacting bone mineralization and blood vessel health.

Natto, a fermented soy food high in MK-4 is popular in certain regions of Japan. Elderly women living in those regions who eat natto have higher bone density than non-natto-eaters. Older men who consume the highest amounts of natto have higher bone density than men who consumed little.

Because bone and blood vessel health are concerns for older people, researchers are investigating whether this form of K will be beneficial. Since natto is an acquired taste to say the least, supplements of menaquinone might be helpful. The research is ongoing.

Meanwhile supplement companies are on the vitamin K bandwagon. Many multiple vitamins for older adults now include some vitamin K2, and you can also buy menaquinone supplements.

Should you? The jury is not yet in. If K2 shows potential for enhancing bone strength and lowering risk for blood vessel calcification, K2 supplementation might gain importance for people with osteoporosis or cardiovascular disease. Because, realistically, few people are going to become natto eaters. There's a complication for many people who are taking anticoagulants. Some of those medications work by interfering with vitamin K, in which case adding more vitamin K as a supplement might be a bad idea.

So that's the current state of information on vitamin K. If you eat a balanced diet with plenty of green vegetables, you are not likely to need a vitamin K1 supplement. And you should be eating a diet like that for a lot of other reasons. As for K2, I'm not going to say one way or the other whether you should take a supplement. It's a very interesting vitamin, a perfect example of the fact that there's always something new in nutritional science, and we should keep open minds. If you have osteoporosis and someday your doctor suggests a vitamin K2 supplement, now you know why.

Iron

"I'm feeling tired. I must need some iron."

This is a common but wrong way to decide to take an iron supplement. The mineral iron is one nutrient most older adults do *not* need to take as a supplement. Post-menopausal women are no longer losing significant amounts of iron every month, so iron status is more stable. And we do get iron from many foods. The form of iron in meat, fish and poultry is well absorbed. Eggs, plant foods and fortified foods contain iron salts, which are less well absorbed.

It's estimated that an older adult needs to absorb about 1-2 mg of iron per day to cover normal iron losses. Unless you are losing significant blood as a result of some medical condition or have been diagnosed with iron deficiency anemia, a daily intake of 8 mg of iron per day from various food sources will cover your needs, as only a small percentage is actually absorbed. It's fairly easy to consume that much from a balanced diet, especially if you are not vegan or vegetarian.

Excess iron in tissues can be toxic and lead to metabolic problems. Normally, iron absorption is controlled by a complex set of regulator molecules. Some people have a hereditary condition – hemochromatosis -- that interferes with this regulation. Iron builds up in tissues, leading to can build up in your body, causing metabolic problems.

Ironically, some of the symptoms of iron overload mimic symptoms we commonly associate with iron deficiency: fatigue and weakness. This is why it's very important to be assessed for chronic fatigue that interferes with your quality of life. Self-diagnosing with iron deficiency and taking a supplement could backfire.

Even if you're post-menopausal, you could still develop iron deficiency if your diet is poor, or you have absorption problems due to other medical problems. Diagnosis of iron deficiency is fairly straight-forward. If you do have that, your doctor will likely recommend a supplement.

There are several forms of supplemental iron to choose from

- Sulfate
- Fumarate
- Gluconate
- Bisglycinate
- Complexes of peptides, amino acids and saccharides

Ferrous sulfate may be the most common form, but it's known to cause stomach upset for some people. A form called heme-iron polypeptide appears to be the best absorbed. If you are advised to take iron to correct a deficiency, your physician will have specific recommendations for you. Do not take excess doses, as iron can cause toxicity problems.

Take Away: Older women need much less iron than women in child-bearing years. While iron deficiency is less likely with age, it isn't unheard of. Simply feeling fatigued isn't a reason to load up on iron supplements. This needs to be diagnosed properly with blood tests. Deficiency could be caused by chronically poor intake or a medical condition, in which case a supplement may be recommended.

Omega-3 fats

Unless you've been living under a rock, you've at least heard of omega-3 fats, also known as fish oil. According to a 2012 survey by the National Center for Complementary and Integrative Health, fish oil was the #1 supplement used by adults in the US. We tend to use the terms fish oil and omega-3 fats interchangeably, but they are not necessarily equivalent. Omega-3 fatty acids are found in fish oil, but they are also found in other foods. Increasingly they are being derived from algae.

As noted in previous chapters, omega-3 fatty acids are biologically unique molecules that perform many very important functions. They play key roles in immunity, brain and eye health and health of blood vessels and cell membranes. Your body cannot synthetize these. They must be consumed.

The "3" refers to the location of the first double bond on the molecule's carbon chain. Omega-6 fats, such as linoleic, have that first double bond in a different location, which makes the molecule a very different shape. And when it comes to molecular structures, form dictates function. Two specific omega-3 fatty acids are biologically active in humans:

1. Eicosapentaenoic acid (EPA) a 20-carbon fatty omega-3 acid
2. Docosahexaenoic Acid (DHA), a 22 carbon omega-3 fatty acid

EPA and DHA are found in fatty fish, like salmon, sardines, herring and mackerel. White-fleshed low fat fish have very little omega-3, if any. Some plant foods have significant amounts of a less biologically active form of omega-3 fat, called alpha linolenic acid (ALA). Walnuts, flax, canola oil and chia seeds are the best examples. But the ability of humans to convert the ALA to EPA or DHA is limited.

There is no official daily recommendation for omega-3 intake in the USA. The "Adequate Intake" is 1.1 grams per day for adult women, of which only 10% needs to be EPA/DHA (just 110 mg total). Other countries and organizations have different intake recommendations. Here are a few examples:

Organization/country	Daily Omega-3 recommendation
WHO	1-2 % of total energy
Dept Health/Aging Australia	90 mg DHA/EPA total
European Food Safety Auth	250 mg EPA/DHA total
AFFSA/France	500 mg EPA/DHA total
Nordic Council of Ministers	1% of energy
Academy of Nutrition & Dietetics	500 mg EPA/DHA total
Japan Ministry of Health	>1800 mg EPA/DHA/day for women>70 yrs 2100 mg for women 50-69

Wow, Japan! Keep in mind, in Japan the daily intake from a fish-rich diet is already high, accounting for much of that recommendation. Supplements may be entirely unnecessary there.

What does 1-2% of energy come to? If you're eating roughly 1500 calories/day, that means 15-30 calories from omega-3 fats, or 1.7 to 3.2 grams/day total, higher than the US "Adequate Intake" of 1.1 grams for adult women.

The standard advice to eat fish twice a week might provide you significant omega-3 from food if you actually do eat a fatty fish twice a week, forever. That's a lot of salmon.* Many people aren't going to do that for a lot of different reasons. They also might not be inclined to eat requisite amounts of flax or chia seed or walnuts every single day. Solution: supplements.

As the health benefits (and promises) of omega-3 have become more apparent over the past several years, supplements have taken off. What are the issues?

- **Dose:** Omega-3 supplement dosages are all over the map. You need to look for the section on the label that states "XXX mg EPA, XXX mg DHA", typically at the bottom. A supplement with a total of 300-500 mg omega-3 is a reasonable choice for general health purposes.
- **Quality:** Two distinct forms of fats are used for omega-3 supplements: triglycerides and ethyl esters.
  - Triglycerides are the form of fat found naturally in all food. Basically it's a glycerol backbone with three fatty acids attached. In the case of an omega-3 supplement, those fatty acids would be omega-3s. Our bodies digest triglycerides every time we eat a meal that contains any fat, and there is evidence this form of omega-3 supplement is better absorbed.
  - Ethyl Esters are synthetic fats, not found in nature. Each molecule has two omega-3 fatty acids attached. The benefit is they're cheaper

to manufacture than triglyceride omega-3 supplements.

- You will not find information about the form of omega-3 on the label, unless a manufacturer chooses to disclose that. If you buy for price, you'll likely be buying ethyl ester omega-3 supplements. But if you buy a more expensive product, you might still be getting ethyl esters. The only way to know is if the manufacturer makes a point of informing consumers about their formulation. Typically the ones that do are using the more expensive triglyceride formulation.

- **Source:** fish liver, fish bodies (everything from salmon to anchovies to calamari), krill and algae are common sources. At the moment, only DHA can be obtained from algal sources, and it's best to get both EPA and DHA if you're taking a supplement, as they have different functions. A supplement with just DHA will not be as beneficial. Krill oil is from krill, which is harvested from the ocean by giant factory ships. Krill is the basis of the marine food chain. Everything from fish to penguins to whales depend on this chain. I personally never, ever buy krill oil products because I don't want to contribute to disruption of the marine food chain. Other than that, there is no evidence that omega-3 from one source or another is better absorbed or more effective.

- **Burps!** Some people experience fishy 'repeats' from fish oil capsules. This might be an individual issue, or it might depend on the supplement. You can buy enteric coated pills that prevent that effect. Some capsules are now enhanced with flavors like lemon to mediate any fish burps. One note of caution: unpleasant fishy aftereffects could be caused by rancid capsules. Fish oil supplements in capsules are subject to rancidity from improper storage. Keep them out of light and heat, preferably refrigerated. Don't buy products that have been displayed in a location subject to excessive heat or sunlight.

I've been taking omega-3 for many years. While I started taking them for a specific problem, I've continued for the sake of general health, since I don't eat fish that often.

Take Away: As noted in previous chapters, omega-3 fatty acids are nutrients, important for brain function, eye health, immune function and other health concerns of older women. If you are a dedicated fish eater, especially fatty fish, supplements might be unnecessary. If you do opt for omega-3 supplements, take them with food, preferably a meal with some fat, to enhance absorption. If you're spending money on supplements, you might as well get your money's worth by optimizing absorption. Don't take them on an empty stomach.

*While salmon is typically assumed to be high in omega-3, in fact that will depend on what the salmon ate. Some salmon may have very little omega-3, but there's no way to know.

Vitamin C (ascorbic acid)

To some extent, the entire era of supplements may have started with vitamin C. When Linus Pauling proposed that large doses of vitamin C could cure or prevent diseases, the modest amounts of vitamin C in foods started to sound inadequate. If you're trying to consume 1000 or 2000 mg per day, you can't drink 20 glasses of orange juice. Every. Day. Indefinitely.

Despite the fact that research has mostly failed to prove the promise of cures or disease prevention, vitamin C is still widely available in megadose pills. Obviously someone is buying that stuff.

The vitamin C RDA for older women is a very modest 75 mg/day. A recent review of intakes in different countries suggested 115 mg/day was more appropriate. But nowhere near the 1000-2000 mg or even higher doses you can find in pills.

Vitamin C is water soluble, and excess is immediately flushed out of your system. The Tolerable Upper Limit for intake is 2000 mg/day. But other research suggests that any amount above 250 mg per day is quickly eliminated. So why take more than that?

If you take a multiple, you get some vitamin C from that, but amounts vary. You could be getting that 250 mg, or just the RDA or something in between. If you consume high vitamin C foods (and you should because they're loaded with other nutrients and fiber) you might be getting plenty from food. For the foods listed below, one average serving could cover your RDA for vitamin C:

- Citrus: oranges, grapefruit, tangerines
- Tomatoes
- Peppers
- Broccoli
- Strawberries
- Pineapple
- Papaya
- Brussels sprouts
- Potatoes
- Cabbage
- Kale

Most other fruits and many vegetables also contain some vitamin C. So again, a supplement may be unnecessary.

Take Away: Vitamin C supplements remain popular despite lack of evidence that it cures the common cold, prevents cancer or cures heart disease. If you do take one, don't expect it to work miracles. Vitamin C is a nutrient, not a drug.

Vitamin E

Vitamin E was another popular alleged cure-all vitamin back in the late 20th Century. It was supposed to prevent heart disease and cancer, and supplements with large doses were widely available. Then scientists started doing studies to investigate these assumptions and found some surprising results. In fact for some people, larger doses of vitamin E were linked to *increased* risk for some cancers, prostate cancer in particular.

Aside from those unexpected findings, vitamin E in large doses was not found to be helpful for heart disease, inflammation, hot flashes, wound healing or cataracts. High dose supplements have been linked to increased risk for hemorrhagic stroke, not entirely surprising since vitamin E has anticoagulant properties.

The RDA is 15 mg (22 IU) of alpha-tocopherol, which is the most active form of E. An IU of alpha-tocopherol equals 0.67 mg, and varies slightly for other forms of the vitamin. Single vitamin E supplements are typically much higher than the RDA. Vitamin E is a fat soluble vitamin, and usually supplements are sold as gel caps, and should be taken with a meal that includes fat.

Foods high in vitamin E includes nuts, seeds and the oils made from those. You could meet your recommended intake with 2 TB of peanut butter. Wheat germ and avocados are also good sources.

Take Away: Vitamin E is included is multiples at varying doses. It's also included in many eye health formulas. You'll already be getting supplemental E if you're taking any of those, so an additional vitamin E supplement would be unnecessary, unless there is a specific medical reason. If you're on anti-coagulants, vitamin E could interfere with those, so discuss supplementation with your physician

B Complex and B vitamins

Lumping all the so-called "B" vitamins together into a group is a bit misleading. While these vitamins do frequently function together in metabolic reactions, they can also act alone in other reactions. Plus the food sources vary considerably. B12 is only found in animal-sourced foods while folate is only found in plant foods. But B1 and B2 can come from either. White wheat flour in the US is fortified, by law, with B1, B2, niacin (B3) and folic acid (folate).

The list of B vitamins includes:
- B1 – thiamin
- B2 – riboflavin
- Niacin, sometimes called B3
- Pantothenic Acid sometimes called B5
- B6 – pyruvate
- Biotin (B7)
- Folate (folic acid) sometimes called B9
- B12 - cobalamin

Because we refer to B vitamins as a group, supplement companies have latched on to that concept, producing B complex supplements that contain several, or all, of the B's. Recommended daily intakes are quite low. For example just 1.1 mg/day for B1 (thiamin). Yet B complex supplements typically contain vastly higher doses. You might find "B 50" products, with 50 mg of everything, even though you don't need 50 mg of any of them. But 50 sure sounds good, along the lines of "if a little is good, more is better". A *lot* more. Ask yourself this: if your car needs 6 quarts of oil to run properly, will it run better if you dump 100 gallons of oil over the engine?

B complex supplements are sometimes referred to as stress formulas, as if huge doses of B vitamins somehow alleviate stress. There is zero evidence for that, although it might put more stress on your kidneys getting rid of all the excess B vitamins.

You can buy single supplements of many common B vitamins, such as B1, B2, B6, folate and B12. B12 actually is of special concern to older adults, and is discussed below. The other B's are typically included in multiples at more reasonable doses, equal to or close to the recommended intake.

Recently research has uncovered evidence for adverse effects of high dose B6 supplementation. So-called pyridoxine toxicity can cause numbness, tingling or weakness in the limbs and balance problems. Because those symptoms are also associated with certain nutrient deficiencies and diseases, a person might be tempted to self-medicate with supplements, possibly making the problem worse. One study found that women taking anywhere from 50 mg to 1000 mg/day of B6 developed symptoms that did not resolve a year after they stopped the excess intake. This is especially concerning because B6 is a popular ingredient in B-complex and stress supplements, as well as energy drinks. You could be consuming excessive amounts without realizing it.

Take Away: Unless you have some unusual medical condition that necessitates taking a single B vitamin supplement, you don't need any of those. Taking mega-dose B complex supplements is equally unnecessary. They do not alleviate effects of stress or prevent stress or fix any diseases. If you take a multiple, you are getting most of the B vitamins, depending on how complete the supplement formula is. Some multiples are best described as semi-multiple. See Chapter 13 on Multiples for more information.

Vitamin B12 -- Cyanocobalamin

Vitamin B12 is of particular concern as we age. It's a large molecule and is absorbed by way of a special transporter system called Intrinsic Factor (IF). Before IF can work, B12 must be separated from food in the stomach, by way of stomach acid. Unfortunately, acid secretion decreases with age, so B12 absorption goes down. The same problem results when people take medications to decrease stomach acid. An estimated 30% of adults over age 60 are B12 deficient.

It's not just about dietary intake or absorption. Many medical conditions can contribute to B12 deficiency:
- Parasitic infection
- Certain intestinal surgeries
- Prolonged malabsorption due to illness that affects the digestive system. This can be significant, and may be overlooked by physicians more concerned with treating the disease.
- Crohn's disease or ulcerative colitis
- Gastric bypass surgery

- Alcoholism
- There is new evidence that metformin, a drug used for Type 2 diabetes, can also adversely impact B12 status

One classic but less common reason for B12 deficiency is pernicious anemia. Fans of *Downton Abbey* may remember a character who was diagnosed with this genetic disorder late in the show. With pernicious anemia, the IF transport system does not function, and no B12 is absorbed. Before the B12 molecule was isolated, there was no treatment for this progressively debilitating disease, and people died prematurely from it. It is not a disease of aging, as it can affect young people. The standard treatment has been B12 injections, but recently experts concluded that large oral doses from supplements work too, by way of passive diffusion.

B12 is found only in animal-sourced foods like meat or eggs, so intake may decline if people consume fewer of these foods, due to taste changes, chewing difficulty, convenience or cost. Vegans of any age are at risk for B12 deficiency because they consume no animal foods.

The B12 is food is bound to protein, and must first be detached from that protein, by way of stomach acid, before it can be absorbed. The form of B12 used in supplements and food fortification is not bound to protein, and so is more readily absorbed. This means supplements may be more useful for older adults who have less stomach acid.

B12 is included in multiples, and senior multiples tend to have higher doses. Some are two hundred or more times the RDA. That big number sounds alarming, but there's a reason: if the IF transport system isn't working and stomach acid is insufficient, the only other way to absorb B12 is by passive diffusion from intestines into blood. That's a very inefficient method, so only a very small portion of the big dose – only about 1% -- ever gets into your system. You can also find single B12 supplements, and they typically are high dose for this reason.

Why would you take B12? Some doctors believe all older

people should have some supplemental B12 because of declining absorption. B12 is involved with many critical functions, including brain function, nerve function, DNA synthesis, red blood cell production and possibly bone mineralization.

How would you know if you were deficient? Well, there are blood tests, but simply testing for B12 might not give a complete picture or your status. According to the National Library of Medicine, the normal range for B12 is 200 to 900 picograms* per milliliter. A blood level of less than 200 pg/ml is a sign of deficiency, but older adults may have deficiency symptoms with levels between 200 to 500 pg/ml.

B12 is necessary for metabolism of homocysteine and methylmalonic acid (MMA), two substances implicated in risk for cardiovascular disease. A B12 value in that 200-500 pg/ml range might look OK to a doctor, but it should be followed up with an MMA test. Elevated MMA means insufficient B12 even if the B12 value appears to be in the normal range. Another catch for some people: liver or kidney disease can interfere with B12 analysis and give a falsely high value. So as you can see, it's not a simple deficiency to diagnose. Studies show that MMA and a related metabolite – homocysteine – are elevated before blood levels of B12 fall into the deficiency range. Some experts believe MMA and homocysteine are better indicators of B12 status.

For older adults, the neurological effects of B12 deficiency could be mistaken for something else. Consider this list:

- Cognitive impairment
- Abnormal gait, awkwardness
- Irritability
- Peripheral neuropathies (numbness, tingling, burning)
- Weakness and loss of balance

Certainly all these problems could have other causes, and easily be ignored by a physician. Some people might just write them off to "getting old". Yet there could be a simple solution –

increased B12.

One other classic sign of severe B12 deficiency is megaloblastic anemia, or enlarged red blood cells. Unfortunately, this symptom can be masked by high folate intake, and it may be one of the last symptoms to emerge, by which time you're already experiencing neurological problems.

So while outward symptoms may certainly provide clues, it's hard to officially diagnose a deficiency without a number of blood tests. Should you take a supplement without an official diagnosis, or without even doing lab tests? Some physicians and organizations recommend a B12 supplement for people over 50. The Linus Pauling Institute recommends 100-400 micrograms/day. There is no official Tolerable Upper Intake limit set, because risk for toxicity is low thanks to poor absorption.

I actually had a problem with B12 awhile ago due to a malabsorption issue, so started taking it. Now, I may take it 2-3 times a week now, just to be sure I'm covered. My blood levels remain within the normal range.

Take Away: In my professional opinion, I think all older adults, perhaps from age 55 on, should be screened periodically for B12 status. Maybe only once every 2-5 years. Certainly you should be screened if you have any of the risk factors, or are taking medications known to interfere with stomach acid.

If you experience some of the symptoms linked to B12 deficiency, you should discuss testing with your doctor. Some physicians believe any older adult with significant cognitive impairment or dementia should be screened for B12. There is evidence that some people with dementia have low B12, which could be contributing to, or causing, the problem.

*A picogram is one trillionth of a gram, or a millionth of a microgram, a very small amount.

Magnesium

This mineral isn't usually on the supplementation radar screen, but perhaps it should be. Magnesium intakes from food are typically below recommendations, even for younger people. Aging has its own negative effects:

1. decreased absorption
2. increased loss through kidneys
3. decreased intake due to diet changes

Other potentially negative impacts on magnesium status come from alcohol intake, medications commonly used by older adults and malabsorption caused by disease.

Magnesium impacts bone health, energy metabolism, protein synthesis, blood pressure and heart health. Poor magnesium status has also been linked to increased risk for migraines, asthma and type 2 diabetes. All of these problems are more common as we age. The connection to bone health is especially important. We're told to take calcium, but magnesium is also critical for bone mineralization.

The best food sources include:

- Whole grains
- Nuts
- Greens like spinach
- Legumes

The daily recommended intake for older women is 320 mg/day. You could consume that much from 4 *cups* of cooked spinach or 1 cup peanut butter (1500 calories!) or 5-1/3 cups cooked black beans or 14 slices 100% whole wheat bread or 10 bananas. Or some combination of those sorts of foods, every single day. Who is going to eat that much? People on a vegan or vegetarian diet might come close.

You can see the dilemma. Your appetite and energy needs are lower than they were 30 years ago, yet you still need the same intake of magnesium. The result of chronic low intake isn't likely to be outright magnesium deficiency, but rather chronic poor magnesium status. It's not something doctors test for, despite the fact that low magnesium is linked to many of the chronic diseases that are common these days, including osteoporosis. A supplement might be appropriate.

Like all minerals, too much isn't a good thing. Most magnesium supplements are 250 mg or less. Multiples might have as much as 100 mg per daily dose, usually less. If you take a daily multiple with 100 mg, you might not need any more supplemental magnesium. If you don't take a multiple and aren't a big consumer of greens, nuts, legumes and whole grains, you could consider a separate magnesium supplement.

Some medical conditions and medications can interact with magnesium, so if you are taking daily medications you should ask the prescribing doctor about those interactions. Magnesium can interfere with some drugs, while other drugs can interfere with magnesium.

Take Away: Barring some unusual medical condition, a supplement with 250 mg or less of magnesium is plenty for most people who want to make up for low dietary intake. Another strategy is to take it every other day while adding more of those higher magnesium foods to your diet. Take any magnesium with food, not on an empty stomach. If you take a multiple, check the label for magnesium content, as that amount might be sufficient.

Zinc

The mineral zinc is a major player in immune function. Low blood levels are linked to increased risk for pneumonia, prolonged infections and more use of antibiotics. We don't need much zinc, compared to other minerals like calcium or magnesium, but we do need enough.

The recommended daily intake for zinc is 8 mg. Our best food sources of zinc are animal-sourced foods, like meat. Oysters are famously high in zinc. You could get your daily requirement from 2 raw oysters. If you aren't a frequent oyster-eater, red meats and poultry and also excellent sources. A modest 4 oz portion of beef has almost twice your daily zinc.

Plant foods, such as whole grains, nuts and legumes, also contain zinc, but they also contain compounds that interfere with absorption of zinc. Vegetarians and vegans who avoid supplements need to up their zinc intake from plant foods by about 50%.

Supporting immune function becomes more important as we age, but some aspects of aging can also interfere with zinc intake or absorption. Decreased appetite means eating less food overall, leading to lower zinc intake. Eating less meat, because of taste, chewing or appetite problems, will also decrease zinc intake.

One problem with zinc, like many minerals, is that lab tests are rarely done, so we are left in the dark about whether we need a supplement. If you're prone to chronic infections and have poor wound healing, you might benefit from a supplement as those are considered to be signs of poor zinc status, especially for older adults.

Zinc is typically included in senior multiples, and you can buy it as a single supplement, or in combination with other minerals. If you're taking a multiple on a regular basis and eating meat, you probably don't need additional zinc supplements.

If you avoid meat and don't take a multiple, you might benefit from a zinc supplement. Many come in large doses – 50 mg – although you can find some with a more reasonable 15 mg. The Tolerable Intake limit for zinc is 40 mg/day, making the 50 mg products look excessive. Like other minerals, zinc is not flushed out of your body on a day to day basis. Taking a higher dose zinc once or twice a week should be sufficient, unless you have some medical reason to take more. A 15 mg supplement every other day would cover your needs as well.

Zinc Lozenges

Zinc lozenges for colds are a recent entry in the nutrition-immunity arena. There's evidence that zinc has some antiviral activity locally in the throat and nasal passages. Chewing and swallowing the lozenge is not helpful. You have to let the zinc lozenge dissolve slowly in your mouth to get the effect.

Several varieties and doses are available. The acetate and gluconate forms of zinc appear to be most effective when used for this purpose. Flavorings like citric acid and the artificial sweetener sorbitol may interfere with zinc activity. If you try zinc lozenges, follow directions on the package, and don't take more than the recommended dose or for a longer period of time.

Take Away:

Getting enough zinc is important, more so as we age, to support immune function. Inadequate intake, impaired absorption and medication interactions are more common as we age and can have adverse impacts on zinc status. If you eat little meat, a supplement that averages 8 mg/day is reasonable. Many senior multiples have that amount of zinc, so additional zinc would not be necessary unless you had a medical reason to take more.

Other nutrients

Plenty of other nutrients are available in single supplement doses, including iodine, phosphorus, biotin, pantothenic acid, potassium, chromium and choline. Many are included in multiples. In most cases, there is no indication that supplementing provides any health benefit.

Some of these nutrients, such as phosphorus and potassium, are widely distributed in food, making supplementation unnecessary. For people with certain medical conditions, such as kidney disease, additional doses of these from supplements could cause serious problems. Potassium supplements are typically limited to 99 mg/pill. Since the daily recommended intake is over 4000 mg, pills could never contribute a meaningful amount.

Chromium is involved in insulin activity, glucose control and energy metabolism. Some health experts developed a theory that supplemental chromium would improve blood glucose and fight Type 2 diabetes. Studies using supplemental chromium for that purpose have not shown any evidence of benefit. Some common medications used by older adults may interfere with chromium absorption, while others may increase it. In any event, there's no evidence that extra chromium, beyond what you might find in a multiple, provides any additional health benefits.

Biotin is sometimes promoted as to prevent hair loss or other quality-of-life benefits. In fact, high doses of biotin can interfere with certain lab tests, leading to false or missed diagnoses.

Iodine is used for thyroid hormone production. It's found in iodized table salt, fish, dairy foods, seaweed and produce grown on soils with significant iodine content. Deficiencies are rare in developed countries. The recommended intake is 150 micrograms/day for an adult; the recommended upper limit is 1100 mcg. Contrary to wishful thinking, taking iodine supplements beyond the daily requirement does not boost metabolism. Excess iodine creates toxic side effects and could lead to interaction with other medications.

Take Away: You can find single supplement products of several other nutrients, but there's no evidence that these provide any health benefit. In some cases, excess intake can have adverse effects. Most of them are included in high quality senior multiple formulas anyway. Of course, at some time in the future, we might find that absorption of one or more of these nutrients decreases with age, and that supplementation is helpful. The following chapter on multiple vitamin/mineral formulas can help you decide if that type of supplement is a better option for you.

13 SUPPLEMENTS – MULTIPLES

Using a term like "multiple vitamin" is a lot like saying "canned soup". There are so many brands and variations, it's impossible to make a blanket statement about them. Here's an important fact: there is no official standard formula for anything labeled "multiple". It's up to the manufacturer to decide what to include and how much.

One thing they all have in common: they include a long list of nutrients. Which nutrients and how much of each is not predictable. The intent is that the consumer – you – thinks the multiple will cover all their nutrient needs. But any multiple that covered all known nutrient needs would be an impossibly large pill. You'd have to divide it into 3-4 pills.

This all begs the question: why take a multiple that covers all known nutrient needs? What about the nutrients in the food you eat? The better formula would cover maybe 30-50% of daily nutrient needs, and truly be a *supplement,* supplementing the nutrients you get from food. What we've got now are more correctly described as *replacements.*

Typical multiples contain:
- Vitamin A: much of it as beta-carotene.
- Vitamin D: most formulas made for seniors (or 50+) now include large doses of vitamin D, up to 1000 IU in some cases. If you already take vitamin D separately, this might end up being too much.
- Vitamin C: the dose can range from 75 mg to 400 or 500.

- Vitamin E: multiples typically don't have high amounts of this.
- B vitamins: these doses can be all over the map. You might find modest RDA amounts for some, but much higher levels for others. Or they're all extremely high. B12 may be present in a large dose due to poor absorption common in older adults, as discussed in the previous chapter.
- Calcium: because calcium salts are bulky, multiples typically don't have high calcium doses, maybe 200 mg.
- Iron: senior/50+ multiples usually omit iron, for reasons discussed in the previous chapter. If you have iron-deficiency anemia, you would need to get iron elsewhere, not from a multiple.
- Zinc: usually present in an amount close to the recommended intake.
- Other minerals like phosphorus, potassium and magnesium may be present in amounts much smaller than the RDA or AI. The form of these minerals can be bulky, so it's hard to include a meaningful dose in a single pill.
- Vitamin K: may be present, especially as a marketing tool, given the new knowledge about bone and vascular health. But some multiples have none.
- Trace minerals like chromium, copper, selenium, manganese, iodine, boron and others may be included. They're called "trace" minerals because only very small amounts are needed every day. Some senior supplements leave many of these out, but I'd recommend finding a formula that did include them.

Other random stuff

Thanks to good PR for antioxidants and lutein, lycopene and other bioactive molecules found in food, supplement manufacturers put token amounts in multiples for the marketing value. Key word: *token*. You can get far more of these from actual food, such as vegetables and fruit.

Exhibit A: lycopene, an antioxidant that's especially concentrated in tomatoes. Some multiples might have 100 µg (micrograms) of lycopene. Sounds impressive? Nope, not when ½ cup of spaghetti sauce has over 23,000 µg. If you want more of this antioxidant, eat some tomatoes or tomato products, preferably as part of a meal that includes some fat, which enhances lycopene absorption.

Choosing Senior Multiples

Find a formula that is as comprehensive as possible. That means it includes the known vitamins and most known minerals, in doses that are not excessive but not so puny as to seem pointless. You can judge how close to the recommended intake each one is using the % DV column. Remember, DV is Daily Value, the recommended intake for someone eating 2000 calories/day. Most older women do not eat that much, although still need the same intake of most vitamins/minerals.

For some of the bulky minerals such as calcium, small percentages are the norm. 100% of recommended intake simply won't fit into one tablet. If you need extra intake of those, you'll probably take a separate supplement.

This table compares the nutrient content of 4 different Senior multiple vitamin/mineral formulas. The "Brand" products are widely available name brands. The column to the right shows the recommended intake for older adult women, so you can see how the products compare to those values.

Some of the formulas have what look like randomly high amounts of some vitamins. Why 4.5 mg of B1? Why 180 mcg of chromium? Because big numbers look good? There seems to be consensus on a few nutrients -- iodine, biotin, folate – which are included in RDA amounts. And none of them have iron, for reasons discussed previously. One has no vitamin E. One has no vitamin K. Why?

By the way, as discussed above, the labels on supplements compare nutrient values to the Daily Value (DV), which is a very general average recommendation based on a 2000 calorie diet. DV does not reflect altered nutrient recommendations for age. So it's better to compare to the RDA for people in our age range.

Nutrient/units	Generic	Brand 1	Brand 2	Brand 3	RDA
Vitamin A IU*	2500	3500	2500	3600	700 mcg
Vitamin C mg	60	100	90	120	75
Vitamin D IU**	1000	1000	1200	1000	15 mcg
Vitamin E IU***	50	35	0	30	15 mg
Vitamin K mcg[1]	30	50	0	20	90
B1 (thiamin) mg	1.5	1.1	1.5	4.5	1
B2 (riboflavin) mg	1.7	1.1	1.7	3.4	1
Niacin mg	20	14	20	20	14
B6 (pyridoxine) mg	2	5	2	6	2
Folate mcg	400	400	400	400	400
B12 mcg	25	50	50	25	2
Biotin mcg	30	30	30	30	30
Pantothenic acid mg	10	5	10	15	5
Zinc mg	11	15	15	24	8
Magnesium mg	50	100	100	50	320
Calcium mg	220	300	500	300	1200
Potassium mg	80	80	0	0	4700
Selenium mcg	19	22	55	27	55
Manganese mg	2.3	2.3	2	4.2	1.8
Chromium mcg	50	52	24	180	20
Iodine mcg	150	150	150	150	150
Copper mg	0.5	0.5	1	2.2	0.9

* The official recommendation for vitamin A intake is now given as micrograms of Retinol Activity Equivalents (RAE). This is intended to avoid confusion about different potency for different forms of vitamin A. Most supplement and food labels still use the old International Unit (IU) measure. The 700 mcg RDA for adult women equals about 2300 IU of preformed active vitamin A, but plant sources of vitamin A are less active, so the IU values for those would be higher. These particular supplements indicate that about 40% of the vitamin A is from beta-carotene, which is half as potent as preformed vitamin A.

** The 15 mcg RDA equals 600 IU of vitamin D.

*** The 15 mg RDA for vitamin E equals 22-23 IU. Supplement companies will have to change their labeling to mcg units in 2018, which will help avoid confusion.

[1] The value for vitamin K is an estimated Adequate Intake, not an official recommended intake. Also this value does not account for

the different forms of K as discussed in Chapter 5. Technically you could consume 90 mcg of only vitamin K1 and assume you had met your requirement.

What's the best choice?

The generic formula referenced in the chart is acceptable. In fact, if you just took it every other day, or took half per day you'd be fine, considering your food also provides all those nutrients and more. You'd be truly *supplementing* your nutrient intake.

But that doesn't mean all generics will have this formula. They're likely to have different formulas. You can do a lot of reading (and squinting at the tiny print on the supplement labels) in the store, or do some research online. Name brand products usually list the nutrients in their multiples, although sometimes the websites make you click through several pages before you find that list.

You can use the following table to enter your own multiple values to compare to the RDA.

Nutrient/units	Your multiple	RDA
Vitamin A (IU)		700 mcg
Vitamin C		75
Vitamin D (IU)		15 mcg
Vitamin E (IU)		15 mg
Vitamin K (AI)		90 mcg
B1 (thiamin)		1 mg
B2 (riboflavin)		1 mg
Niacin		14 mg
B6 (pyridoxine)		2 mg
Folate		400 mcg
B12		2 mcg
Biotin		30 mcg
Pantothenic acid		5 mg
Zinc		8 mg
Magnesium		320 mg
Calcium		1200 mg

Potassium		4700 mg
Selenium		55 mcg
Manganese		1.8 mg
Chromium		20 mcg
Iodine		150 mcg
Copper		0.9 mg
Iron		8 mg

The Interactive DRI webpage is a great tool for people who are curious about the recommended intake for all known nutrients. If you need more information, or want to look up values for trace nutrients, it's a handy resource:

https://www.nal.usda.gov/fnic/interactiveDRI/

What About Gummies

The discussion so far has been about tablets or capsules that you swallow whole. But lately gummy vitamins are all the rage, and they're not just for kids anymore. There's been an explosion in adult gummy vitamin products. I have to wonder why. Perhaps we're reverting to childhood? I've written about gummy vitamins on my blog, and one constant theme is the randomly incomplete formulas.

Unlike tablet multiples, gummies are completely devoid of B1, B2, iron and several other nutrients. A few other nutrients are thrown in, typically in small inconsequential doses. 1% of this, 5% of that. In one case, the dose was 0.01% of the recommended intake, yet there it was in the nutrient listing. What was the point? You probably get more than that just from the water supply.

Why such strangely unbalanced formulas? One likely explanation is that some nutrients do not work well in gummy products. They may cause problems with the structure or flavor or appearance of the gummy candy. They may simply not blend well. The take away in my opinion is that gummy multiples are not a good choice. If you 're going to take a multiple, you should take one that has a comprehensive list of nutrients.

You might prefer gummies because you can't swallow large tablets. In that case you could investigate chewables, which may have better formulas because the chemistry works better. Use the chart above to compare, or check brand name products online first. Another option is to find multiples in smaller tablets. Some companies are making those for this reason. The recommended dose may be 2 per day, which is actually handy. As I've said, taking half a multiple daily should be sufficient in combination with a good diet. If the company has already broken the dose in half, so to speak, so much the better.

TARGETED COMBINATION SUPPLEMENTS

All-purpose multiples take a shotgun approach to nutrition – load every known nutrient into a pill and assume some benefit. The new trend is targeted multiples. As research clarifies the impact of specific nutrients on diseases, supplement companies jump in with targeted formulas of select nutrients. Surveys show that older adults are big users of so-called system-specific supplements, or targeted multiples.

Bone health, vision, menopause and weight loss are some examples of system-specific supplements that might be of interest to older women. Typically the number of nutrients in any of these formulas is limited. In some cases, the doses are far above the recommended daily intake; in other cases not.

Problems could arise if you're taking these types of supplements along with a general purpose multiple and/or single nutrient supplements. You could end up taking excessive amounts of certain nutrients. Many of them, particularly weight and sports/energy supplements, contain other substances like herbs or stimulants that can interact with medications.

Here's another critical point about these targeted supplements: there is no rule that they must be effective. This is an important concept that consumers frequently don't appreciate. The FDA does have jurisdiction over supplement production and labeling, but there is no regulation about whether a supplement *works*. In other words, products labeled "for bone health", "vision support" or "promotes joint strength" may have no effect.

Supplement labels cannot make disease-related claims, such as "prevents macular degeneration" or "treats osteoporosis". At best labels can use pre-approved general statements like "calcium builds strong bones". The label for a national brand of vision supplements says nothing about macular degeneration or the AREDS study. Rather is says "nourish your eyes".

Are targeted multiples useless? Maybe not. But you should use caution if taking one of these along with other types of supplements to avoid excessive intakes of some nutrients.

Vision

The AREDS study, as discussed Chapter 10, measured the potential benefits of a specific nutrient combination on progression of age-related macular degeneration. So-called AREDS supplements are now widely available, with formulas based (sometimes loosely) on the nutrient doses used in the study. As you may remember, the AREDS2 study formula included:

- 500 mg vitamin C
- 400 IU vitamin E
- 10 mg lutein
- 2 mg zeaxanthin
- 350 mg DHA
- 650 mg EPA
- 25 mg zinc
- 2 mg copper

This formula was linked to reduced AMD progression for study subjects, so supplement companies created products to mimic the AREDS nutrient list. They're marketed to support eye health. Strangely, many of the products labeled eye health/AREDS bear little resemblance to the study formula. Here's a comparison of some examples:

Nutrient	AREDS 2	Brand 1	Brand 2*	Brand 3
Vitamin C mg	500	150	250	113
Vitamin E mg	400 IU	20	7.5 IU	100 IU
Zinc mg	25	9	7.5	17.4
DHA mg	350	90	100	125
EPA mg	650	160	0	50
Lutein mg	10	5	10	10
Zeaxanthin mg	2	1	2	2.5

* Brand 2 also includes vitamin A, selenium, resveratrol, copper and fruit powders.

As you can see, the formulas may have some ingredients in common, but the doses seem random and don't always correspond to the original study formula. Not that that's a bad thing. The study formula for AREDS 2 was changed after AREDS 1. In some ways, aside from the lutein and zeaxanthin, the other nutrient values seem random and, especially for vitamins E and C, questionably high.

There a plenty of other vision supplements for sale. Many include vitamin A and other plant extracts and herbs. Some omit copper if the amount of zinc is not too high (copper was originally included to counter the potential interaction with the high dose of zinc). You can also find supplements with only lutein/zeaxanthin, which are after all the key players in macular pigmentation. The AREDS2 formula is especially high in omega-3 fatty acids, which would be unnecessary for people who get omega-3 fats from their diet or from other supplements.

So what should you do about these? If you have a family history of age-related macular degeneration, or you are in early stages of this disease process, increasing intake of lutein and zeaxanthin is a good idea. You could take a supplement, but the better source would be foods, from eggs and avocado to spinach, kale, oranges, peas and corn.

Keep in mind, there is no recommended daily intake of lutein or zeaxanthin. Supplements with up to 10 mg lutein per day appear to be sufficient. Two of the formulas in the chart have 10 mg in a daily dose, as do many others on the market. Whether from food or supplements, these carotenoids should be consumed with a meal that includes fat to enhance absorption.

Another consideration: vision supplements are not cheap. If you already take a multiple, with vitamin E, C and zinc, and you eat plenty of foods high in lutein and zeaxanthin, you might not need extra from a supplement.

Bone Health

Supplement formulas for bone health have expanded beyond simple calcium + vitamin D tablets. As noted in Chapter 5 on bone health, the many other nutrients play key roles in bone structures. There are now numerous specially formulated supplements that claim to "support bone health". What do they contain?

- Calcium: that's a given. But because there are other nutrients in these products, the amount of calcium per tablet may be lower than calcium-only products.
- Magnesium is also important. However it can compete with calcium for absorption, so combining them in one pill is a questionable solution. Most of these supplements have only token amounts of magnesium – maybe 50 mg – much less than the 250 mg you would get in a single magnesium supplement.
- Vitamin D is now standard for bone supplements. And since it's included in other senior-type supplements, you could be taking a lot more than you imagined.
- Vitamin K: K2 plays a role in calcium metabolism and would be appropriate for bone health. Some bone supplements have this vitamin.
- Zinc: this one is a bit of a mystery, as zinc is not known to impact bone mineralization, other than as a nutrient needed for general health.
- Boron: While there is some evidence from animal studies that boron may impact bone mineralization,

there isn't strong evidence that it helps humans build bone.

- Copper: while a deficiency in infants can impact bone integrity, there is no evidence that additional copper is good for bone strength in older adults.
- Manganese: this mineral does play a role in bone and cartilage formation. The recommended intake is 1.8 mg/day. Food sources include nuts and legumes. Raisin bran cereal and pineapple are particularly good sources.
- Strontium: the prescription drug strontium ranelate is a medication used to treat osteoporosis. It has shown some benefit in the treatment of osteoarthritis of the knee. In drug trials, it seems to increase risk for heart attack. The strontium found in supplements is *not this form*, and there is no evidence that the chemical form of strontium found in supplements has any impact on bone structure. Nevertheless, manufacturers of bone supplements rave about the wonders of strontium and include it in supplements.
- Small amounts of other random minerals such as silicon and vanadium.

Strangely, most have no phosphorus or potassium, both of which are known to be very important for bones. Both are required in large amounts every day, so it's likely the supplement manufacturers don't think they can get enough of either into a pill to make a difference. And of course, no pill is going to do much for your protein intake, protein being another critical piece of the bone strength puzzle.

One thing many of these have in common: the manufacturers cherry pick some research data to justify putting trace amounts of various minerals in bone supplements. The research results may come from animal studies, or the results may not have shown much significance, yet that's enough to sprinkle some extra mineral powder into the bone supplement mix so that the Nutrition Facts panel will have an impressively long list of ingredients.

Many of these products brag about using plant or algae-sourced minerals, or chelated minerals. There is no solid evidence that these forms are any better than Plain Jane calcium or magnesium salts.

If you search for "bone supplements" on the web, you'll get millions of results. The first several pages will be cheerful positive reviews from companies making or selling these products, along with 5 star glowing testimonials claiming the supplements worked wonders.

When it comes to bone strength, the ONLY way to assess whether something – diet, supplements, medications – improved your bones is with a DEXA scan. So if you buy a bone health supplement, you won't have any idea if it's helping unless you happened to start taking that supplement immediately after a bone scan that showed thinning bones. In order to truthfully evaluate the bone supplement, you can't do anything else differently -- no medications, no diet changes, no other supplements, no increased exercise, etc. If, after faithfully taking that supplement for 2 or more years, your next bone scan showed improvement, then it's possible the supplement helped you.

Take Away

So-called bone supplements frequently duplicate nutrients found in other products, such as garden-variety multiples. If you need to help your bones, you need to ensure adequate intake of a variety of nutrients, as outlined in the bone health chapter, particularly protein, calcium, phosphorus, potassium, vitamin D and magnesium.

If you're using a supplement to boost calcium and vitamin D intake, you can consume sufficient amounts of other bone nutrients from a nutrient-dense diet. With that in mind, supplements that target only bone health are probably unnecessary and are unlikely to include protein, phosphorus and potassium. Those three key nutrients must come from food.

Joints

Oh those aching knees! Or hips, or [fill in the blank with other joints]. It's an unfortunate part of aging: our joints aren't as supple as they once were. Years of wear and tear, as well as general deterioration associated with aging can cause pain that impedes activity, creates stress and affects quality of life.

There are dozens of possible causes for joint pain, ranging from cancer to rare diseases to injury and arthritis. Aches and pains frequently come and go, and we can recognize situations that may have caused temporary problems, such as improper lifting or overuse during a sport. Sometimes rest and anti-inflammatories are all you need. Chronic nagging joint pain that doesn't improve, or gets worse, should be evaluated by a physician.

Arthritis is a popular target for joint supplements. The primary components of these are chondroitin and glucosamine, neither of which are nutrients. Rather, both are structural components of cartilage. The rationale for taking them is simplistic: the chondroitin and glucosamine you take are absorbed and travel in the blood to your cartilage, helping to repair it.

Study results of benefits have been mixed at best. A review published in 2017 concluded that joint supplements provided moderate short term pain relief, but long-term follow up showed no significant lasting improvements. Nevertheless many people swear by these products.

So far, nutrients have not been identified that specifically relieve joint pain or prevent or slow arthritis. Omega-3 fatty acids has shown promise for pain and morning stiffness associated with rheumatoid arthritis and osteoarthritis, thanks to the anti-inflammatory effect.

Perhaps the most important nutrition-related intervention has nothing to do with supplements: weight loss. If you're obese or significantly overweight, your joints are under more stress and more prone to injury and overuse. Regular exercise, part of any healthy lifestyle, helps to strengthen muscles that support those joints.

Take Away:

Joint supplements typically do not involve nutrients. Chondroitin and glucosamine are popular ingredients, but are not nutrients. Claims for benefits are made for a variety of herbal products and food extracts as well.

In the future, medical technology will certainly give us more treatment choices, such as personalized joint replacement parts or specialized injections. Meanwhile, the best first line defense for joints is normal body weight and regular physical activity.

Weight Supplements

Dieters are always looking for the magic elixir that's going to melt fat effortlessly. Weight loss supplements appeal to that magical belief. They're among the most popular supplements and also responsible for ¼ of emergency room visits related to supplements.

Common ingredients include caffeine, green tea extracts, some B-vitamins and perhaps cayenne pepper extract. Caffeine is a stimulant and can help suppress appetite. Cayenne pepper and green tea may encourage cells to burn more fat, although the effect is small. Random B-vitamins are added because they're involved with energy metabolism, except consuming excess amounts does not boost metabolism.

Other ingredients come and go depending on research and marketing. Most are herb or food extracts. Unfortunately many weight loss supplements are found to contain undeclared prescription drugs, which could be dangerous. Note the above reference to emergency room visits due to dietary supplements.

Take Away:

Given the worsening obesity epidemic, do you imagine that a supplement that actually caused quick effortless weight loss would remain a secret? If any of these actually worked, why do we still have an obesity epidemic? Think about that if you're ever tempted to buy a weight loss supplement.

Appearance Supplements

Remember when eating gelatin desserts was supposed to give you beautiful finger nails? That mid-20th Century advice never panned out, although it probably helped make Jello popular. Decades later, nails, skin and hair are still a concern, and we still have nutritional advice on how to improve them. Trouble is, the advice isn't all that useful.

Obviously skin, hair and nails are part of your body, and various nutrients are essential for them to grow and maintain integrity. Key word "nutrients". There is no one nutrient that controls the growth of any of these.

Take fingernails. They're made of a special protein called alpha-keratin, the same component of animal hooves. Adequate quality protein from your diet is important for healthy nails, but the growth process depends on many other nutrients as well. Deficiencies of iron and vitamin C are known to impact nail health. There's evidence that low magnesium also affects nails. Recently biotin supplements have been promoted to fight brittle nails. The key point is that deficiencies of some nutrients can affect nail health. If you aren't deficient, and your nails are otherwise healthy, taking extra doses of nutrients won't help.

Hair is made of the protein keratin. Like fingernails, hair is actually dead once it grows out of the scalp. Hair grows more quickly than fingernails, and can more quickly show the impact of a generally poor diet. Malnutrition at any age is associated with dry, dull, stringy hair that falls out more easily. Prolonged dieting using unbalanced diets, anorexia, famine and poor food intake due to illness can all impact hair. As with nails, the problem isn't one nutrient; it's the whole diet.

Skin is a far more complex structure than hair or nails. Skin grows from the inside out, and the different layers have different physical properties. As we age, the lower support layers lose elasticity. The outer layer turns over more slowly. Skin becomes more fragile, dull and saggy. External factors like sun exposure, smoking and environmental pollutants can exacerbate the process.

Because skin is so complex, it's hard to pin point nutrients that are more important than others for skin health. Protein and fats are important for skin structure and growth. Vitamins A, C, D and E, as well as minerals such as zinc, play key roles in maintaining skin structure and integrity. Adequate intakes of these are important. Deficiencies can adversely impact skin, but excessive intakes won't make your skin better.

Acne isn't just for teenagers. Older women can get it too. Plenty of foods are blamed for acne – chocolate being the most well-known --, and you may have your own list of offending foods, but recent research suggests that the skin's microbial community is also a factor. It's not that your skin should be antiseptic. It's that the wrong bacteria can set you up for spots. The relationship between acne and diet is not clear, and certainly it varies from one person to another. A dermatologist or skin care expert can help you with advice on general skin care, you'll have to pay attention to how your skin responds to foods you eat. My problem food: dairy fats, particularly butter. Sigh!

Age alone impacts skin, hair and nails, regardless of your nutrient intake. The question is: can a stellar diet lessen the effects of aging? There isn't any solid evidence, but that doesn't stop supplement companies from developing so-called Hair-Skin-Nails supplements.

The formulas for some of these products read like your basic multi vitamin: B vitamins, A,C,D,E, a few minerals such as zinc and magnesium. There may be small amounts of herbs and food extracts. For most, the key difference is biotin, present at levels that can be 1000%, 1700% and 3500% of the recommended daily intake.

Why so much biotin? The daily recommendation is 30 micrograms. The justification for megadoses is a small study done almost 30 years ago, in which women with brittle nails were given a very large dose of biotin. Why biotin? It was known to help strengthen the hooves of horses. If it helps horses, why not humans? Nail thickness increased modestly in the women who took biotin, so now we have megadoses.

A more recent study of women with hair loss found only a small number had actual biotin deficiency. The study authors rejected the idea that high dose biotin supplementation is a treatment for hair loss.

Nevertheless the belief persists and megadose biotin shows up in these hair/nail/skin supplements. If a little is good, a lot must be better. Or not. Recently the FDA has issued a Safety Communication about these megadose biotin supplements. High biotin in blood interferes with dozens of lab tests, including some that may be critical to life. Thyroid tests are particularly susceptible to this interference, creating false high readings. So you could have low thyroid, but a megadose biotin supplement could skew your lab test to show normal thyroid, and you are not given appropriate treatment.

Take Away:

Special supplements for hair/nails/skin have many nutrients common to multiple vitamins and may have very high doses of biotin. At the moment there is no good evidence that particular nutrients can reverse the normal effects of aging on hair, nails or skin. The best nutritional strategy is a really good diet, along with avoidance of environmental stressors like sun and smoking.

Natural Sunscreen?

Carotenoids, those fat-soluble pre-vitamin A antioxidants found in vegetables and fruit, are known to accumulate in skin, where they appear to have photoprotective activity. Several studies have demonstrated some degree of protection from UV damage in skin that was enriched with carotenoids by supplementation. While the carotenes from carrots and sweet potatoes aren't a substitute for a good sunscreen, they can help protect your skin from damage. Just another really good reason to load your diet with dark-colored vegetables and fruit

Summing Up Multiples

Predictions:
1. Disease-specific combination supplements are the wave of the future. We will undoubtedly see a proliferation of these products.
2. All-purpose multiples will stick around, increasingly sprinkled with a token dusting of food or herb extracts with impressive-sounding names.

One potential problem of the growth in targeted supplements is nutrient overlap and excessive intakes. While your kidneys can flush out excess water soluble substances, fat-soluble nutrients stick around. Vitamins A and D can accumulate over time, leading to toxicity symptoms. Minerals can also accumulate to toxic levels. For example, excess zinc interferes with copper, so if you're getting zinc from a multiple and an eye formula and perhaps a bone or skin formula, you could be overloading on this mineral, and risk developing signs of copper deficit.

You need *sufficient* intakes of nutrients. Excessive intakes will not improve your health, your skin, your hair, your eyes, your bones or make you lose weight. And as we see from the recent biotin problem, excessive intakes of nutrients could cause problems no one anticipated.

Here are some reasons you might consider taking a supplement:

1. Your diet isn't well balanced, or you have a very poor appetite.
2. You're recovering from significant unplanned weight loss caused by illness.
3. You like the idea of a supplement covering all your bases, so to speak, for nutrient intake.
4. You've been advised to take one by your physician.

Here are some reasons you might *not* take a supplement:
1. You just don't like taking pills.

2. You feel that your diet is very good and taking a supplement is a waste of money or simply pointless.
3. You just don't like them (they upset your stomach, or some other reason).
4. You've been advised not to take them by a physician.

This last reason brings up an important consideration that's especially applicable for older adults: drug-nutrient interactions. Prescription medications can interact adversely with nutrients. Nutrients can interfere with drug action; drugs can interfere with nutrient absorption or utilization.

For example, many chemotherapy drugs impede cancer cell growth by interfering with folate metabolism. Taking folate supplements while taking such a drug may decrease drug effectiveness. Calcium can interfere with absorption of thyroid and other medications. Drug information inserts typically include cautions and instructions about known interactions. Your pharmacist will also have that information.

The nutrient interactions apply to nutrients from foods and supplements. You can't always avoid a specific nutrient in food, but you can avoid supplements if necessary. When taking a prescription drug, your pharmacist or physician may warn you against certain supplements. As multiples contain most known nutrients, multiples might present a problem. For example, if you take thyroid medication, and your multiple contains calcium, you should probably avoid taking a multiple close to the time of day you take thyroid.

What I do

I take the idea of *supplementation* seriously. I don't feel I need to get 100% or more of daily nutrient requirements from pills. Food provides significant amounts. I find a general purpose senior-type multiple and break it in half. In fact, I might only take half every 2 days. So on average, the supplement covers 25% of recommended doses of many nutrients. That's fine with me.

When picking a multiple:
- I look for senior-type formulas, typically without iron.
- I don't look for high doses of B vitamins; I stick to RDA-level doses.
- I don't expect to get omega-3 from a multiple.
- I completely don't care about token amounts of antioxidants, lycopene, lutein or similar substances that I'd prefer to get from food.
- I don't care at all about gluten-free or Non-GMO or any other Health Halo marketing gimmicks.

I can usually find a generic version that fits my criteria. Because I'm not being paid to endorse any particular brand, and because brands change their formulas frequently, I'm not recommending anything specific. You can research many brand name supplements on company websites, although sometimes you have to click through several pages in order to find the list of nutrients. Major brands typically are reliable in terms of quality and safety of their products. For the most part, generic versions of brand name formulas are just as reliable.

If you'd prefer to just take a multiple and not be bothered with separate vitamin D or B12, you can find formulas with higher amounts of those key nutrients. You won't find any one multiple that includes significant calcium however, as the chemical form is too bulky for one pill. So if calcium is important to you, you might need a separate supplement.

Resources on supplements

Supplements change all the time. Research on nutrients provides new insights. Doses and formulas are tweaked, new products are developed. Products are found to be adulterated, or not to contain what's listed on the label; warnings are issued. It's impossible to keep current with all of this in a book.

Fortunately there are reliable online resources for people interested in up-to-date information on supplements. Here are some of my Go-To sources:

WebMD Vitamins and Supplements Center
https://www.webmd.com/vitamins-supplements/default.aspx
The WebMD online resource provides information on nutrients and herbs, including metabolic roles and uses and effectiveness for disease processes. For example, a search on "niacin" yields information on how this vitamin works, while a search on "osteoporosis" results in a long list of nutrients, herbs and foods rated from "likely effective" to "insufficient evidence" to "possibly ineffective", accompanied by links to studies. This kind of information is useful to someone who has heard that some herb or nutrient helps a condition, but wants to verify the claim.

Natural Medicines Comprehensive Database
http://naturaldatabase.therapeuticresearch.com/home.aspx
The NMCD is a subscription database, primarily intended for health professionals, but you can obtain some basics without a subscription. The database includes information on nutrients, herbs and food components such as caffeine. You can find data on effectiveness, drug-nutrient interactions and medical conditions.

National Institutes of Health Office of Dietary Supplements
https://ods.od.nih.gov
The National Institutes of Health Office of Dietary Supplements has free consumer-oriented fact sheets on dietary supplements, which includes nutrients, herbs and food components.

U.S. Pharmacopeia
http://www.quality-supplements.org
This website has information about quality and certification issues related to dietary supplements, including use of the USP Verified Mark, which you will find on some supplement products.

Linus Pauling Institute
http://lpi.oregonstate.edu/mic/disease-index
Located at Oregon State University, the Institute maintains a website with detailed information about nutrients and other food components as related to health and disease.

DOD/Operation Supplement Safety
https://www.opss.org
The DOD Uniformed Services University maintains a website aimed at military personnel, but open to anyone. It has basic information as well as up-to-date information about supplement safety, which can be a particular issue for military personnel. Fitness and weight loss products might be of particular interest to older adults.

ConsumerLab
https://www.consumerlab.com
Consumer Lab is a subscription website with a wealth of information about nutrients, herbs, food components and dietary supplement products. CL reviews products for adulterants and verifies doses stated on the label, and issues alerts when products do fail testing. Not all possible products are reviewed however.

There are certainly other resources online, some not so reliable. Don't get your supplement information from a website that is promoting or actively selling the supplement in question, or a rival supplement. The above list gives you plenty of options to find reliable and unbiased information.

14 WEIGHT: LOSING AND GAINING

LOSING

At this point in your life, if you've been an up-and-down serial dieter, you may have reached this conclusion: you're just going to be OK with the weight you've got. Sure you might rather weigh a few pounds less, but it's not worth the effort. If your weight lies somewhere between "normal" and overweight, I'm not going to question your decision. Enjoy life, enjoy food, stop worrying about it.

The only situation that might warrant continued efforts at weight loss is if you are obese, to the point where it interferes with your life. Excess weight can cause joint problems, especially knees, ankles and hips, impacting mobility and stability. And it's a Catch 22 situation: the more your joints hurt, the less mobile you become, and the harder it is to control your weight.

There are many medical reasons to stay out of the obese weight range. You may be familiar with some of these increased risks linked to obesity:

- breast cancer and colon cancer
- Type 2 diabetes
- Hypertension and stroke
- Cardiovascular disease
- Reflux disorder
- Breathing problems
- infections

With weight loss, all of these risks decrease. And it doesn't take a lot of weight loss. Just losing 10% of body weight can quickly improve insulin sensitivity, blood glucose levels, blood pressure and blood cholesterol.

What should you weigh?

A discussion about what you should weigh is loaded with potential conflicts and unintended consequences. When it comes to weight, I'm not going to dictate to anyone in our age group about what the scale should say. Rather, I've got suggestions for helping you decide for yourself.

You've probably heard of BMI, or Body Mass Index. It's a formula developed years ago to try to make numerical sense of normal weight and obesity. It's an imperfect system, but it's what we've got.

BMI is calculated like this: Weight (in kilograms) divided by Height (in meters) squared, or kg/m^2. You can find plenty of BMI calculators online, so you don't have to do the conversion of pounds to kilograms and so forth. The values usually range from 17 to the 40's. You can find one online calculator here: http://www.bmi-calculator.net

According to the NIH, the BMI standard ranges are:

- Underweight: < 18.5
- Normal weight: 18.5 – 24.9
- Overweight: 25 – 29.9
- Obese: 30 and above.

In some cases, there are valid reasons to quibble about the "overweight" range, especially for people who are highly muscled, and so weigh more than a normal weight person, but are not overly fat. However, once BMI rises above 30, it's increasingly hard to argue that your higher weight is due to anything but excess fat.

So you might do the math and find that your current weight is Normal. Fine, right? Not so fast. Lately medical researchers have raised concerns that BMI ranges should be adjusted for post-menopausal women. Why? Because, as mentioned previously, we lose muscle as we age, while gaining fat tissue. You might be in the Normal weight range, but you might actually be over-fat. It's called sarcopenic obesity: as muscle mass is lost with age (sarcopenia), fat mass replaces it. The result is a thin-appearing person who in fact has high body fat, and it's excess body fat, not just weight, that's linked to disease risks.

For research purposes, obesity can also be defined as 35% body fat. Research on post-menopausal women, using a DEXA scan to measure body fat, compared percent body fat to BMI. A significant number of women with BMI less than 30 (the obesity cut off) were in fact obese based on percent body fat. The conclusion was that BMI isn't a foolproof method for classifying older women as obese.

New evidence from a large ongoing study of women's health makes this issue more concerning. Higher percent body fat is linked to increased risk for estrogen-positive breast cancer in post-menopausal women, regardless of actual body weight. The good news from this particular study was that exercise matters. The women with higher body fat percentage exercised less.

What does this mean for you? Do you need a body fat percentage scale or frequent DEXA scans? Well, frequent DEXA scans aren't feasible. You can find home scales that measure body fat, but the measurements aren't as accurate as a scan. They are also more expensive than a no-tricks bathroom scale. They are mainly useful to track change. You might find an inexpensive scale that says your body fat is 29% (even though it might actually be anywhere from 28 to 31%). But if you've embarked on a weight management regimen, and you lose body fat, the scale should be able to show your percentage going down, which is useful and encouraging information.

The easiest strategy would be to keep your weight in the normal range, eat adequate protein as discussed in Chapter 6, and stay active to support muscle mass. The best exercise plan would involve aerobic activities combined with weight or strength training to challenge upper body and core muscles, all of which are susceptible to age-related loss.

Weight Losing Strategies

So you decide you want to lose some weight. But you've

tried everything before, and there's nothing new I can tell you, right? This might be true, but I can at least reiterate what current nutrition knowledge tells us about diets that are associated with both normalized body weight and better health. Whatever you call these diets, they all have some common characteristics:

1. Plant-based. You don't have to be vegan to eat a more plant-based diet. The Mediterranean style diet includes modest portions of meat and dairy foods, and is linked to better weight control, despite allowing for liberal amounts of fat, mostly as vegetable oils (olive oil being the most famous one). Why plant based? Plant foods are loaded with nutrients, and also high water content. They fill you up, creating satiety so you naturally end up eating fewer calories. The Mediterranean style diet also allows for a higher fat intake, making it more satisfying.

2. Sufficient protein. Chapter 6 has plenty of information about protein needs of older adults. Protein also creates satiety, and including adequate protein at *all* your meals helps to turn off your appetite, until the next meal.

3. Moderate fat, particularly from plant sources. Fat makes food taste good and also contributes to satiety. Vegetable oils are preferable to animal fats. Low fat diets are notoriously hard to stick with, and have a poor track record when it comes to long term weight control. While they may work in theory for weight loss, if you can't stick to the diet, then in reality it doesn't work.

4. Room for treats. Don't expect yourself to eat a pristine diet for long. Giving up sugar or carbs or creating rigid food rules never lasts long, and then you feel guilty for not following through on your plan. But keep those treats to a minimum. It may be helpful to avoid keeping tempting foods in your home, because it's too easy to nibble away at them.

For example, the occasional ice cream treat is a cone you buy at an ice cream shop, not a dish you scoop from the half gallon lurking in your freezer (tempting you to go back for seconds and thirds).

Calorie Consciousness

What about counting calories? Calorie counting has been the basis of reducing diets since the beginning of time. Well before calories were defined as a measure of food energy, people understood that, if you were overweight, cutting back on food intake helped to take weight off.

Now calorie counting is enshrined in Western culture. Food labels all contain calorie information. Processed foods are engineered to be lower calorie. Many people religiously track daily calorie intake, turning eating into a math problem. Dieters try to constrain their appetite and food choices to fit the permitted calorie limit. Fitness apps and exercise machines tell us how many calories we've burned, to varying degrees of accuracy. Some dieters use that information to 'eat back' calories they supposedly burned, as a reward for exercising, defeating the purpose of the exercise. Despite all this calorie counting, obesity rates rise.

What do I think of calorie counting? I think it has a place for people who are trying to lose weight, if it helps those people to be more conscious about portion sizes and food choices. But anyone tracking calories has to understand that there is always going to be inaccuracy. You might think you are eating only 1500 calories a day, but in fact you might be eating 1700 some days, or 1450 or whatever. Calorie values for foods are not 100% accurate. Your ability to measure your portion of some food is not always going to be accurate. Eating homemade foods prepared from recipes adds another degree of inaccuracy. Calorie *counting* is not the best description of what's possible. Calorie estimating is more truthful.

Should you track calories? Only if you are trying to lose weight and you feel that being mindful of calories helps you stick to your plan. Simply cutting back on food – limiting portion sizes and servings and eliminating high calorie junk food – can also work, without bothering about the math.

How many calories? You can find lots of websites and apps that calculate recommended calorie levels. Just don't expect any of them to be completely accurate for your situation. Most use one of the energy equations created for diet research. These equations use gender, height, weight, age and other factors to compute the number of calories you would need merely to cover basic energy needs such as heart beat, breathing, cell metabolism and brain function. Then calories burned by physical activity are added to that number. For most of us, the basal number represents most of the calories you burn in a day. For older women, this will range from about 1100 calories for a small-sized person to 1500+ for a very tall and heavy woman. Physical activity might add 20% to 50% more, depending on your activities and level of exertion. Here's one handy website that calculates calories and a number of other parameters:

http://www.bmi-calculator.net/bmr-calculator/

The rule of thumb for weight loss is to eat 500 fewer calories per day, on average, than your total requirement of basal calories + activity calories. If you are consistent at cutting back (key word: consistent), you lose weight, although probably not at a predictable rate due to shifts in body fluids. If you reduced your calorie intake by fewer, say 300 per day, you'd lose weight at a slower pace.

I'm not opposed to calorie counting. Many people find it helpful. Just don't expect it to be 100% accurate. It's still about eating less food. If you are counting calories for weight loss, and you don't lose weight, then your counts are not very accurate.

What about diet trackers?

Food and diet trackers are becoming increasingly popular and accessible as phone and tablet apps. If you need an extra level of self-monitoring, a tracker might be useful. You can get information on calories, protein, fat and most known nutrients. The problem is you have to take the time to enter the foods you ate, as accurately as possible. You might not always remember exact portions sizes, or might misjudge them. You might not be able to find a listing for the exact food you ate. Or you might find a listing, but the data for that food is inaccurate. That said, they can at least tell you if you're in the ballpark for your calorie or nutrient goals. Trackers have their uses, but are not foolproof.

When I counsel people about weight loss, I usually look for all the different ways a person might be packing excess calories into the day. Common examples include:

- Alcoholic drinks, especially fancy cocktails or beer
- Snacks
- High calorie coffee or tea drinks every day
- Late evening/after dinner eating
- Large portions/second helpings
- Habitual mindless eating while watching TV, driving, etc.
- High calorie side dishes at meals
- Eating out of containers, not from a plate or bowl.

None of these choices are necessary, but they can easily become comfortable habits that brighten your day. If you're trying to lose weight and keep it off, and you recognize any of these, you're going to have to think about that. How important are comfortable enjoyable habits compared to weighing less? How important are comfortable habits compared to health risks? Usually eliminating, or restricting, those calorific food habits is sufficient to help you cut back without really thinking about numbers. If you just ate 3 meals that were a reasonable size, you'd probably be fine.

A comfortable habit run amok

For several months a few years ago, I couldn't help noticing that an acquaintance had been losing some serious weight. I asked her what changes she'd made, and she emphatically responded "Gave up sugar." She'd gotten into the habit of treating herself to a sweet snack every afternoon. Then the modest sweet snack morphed over time into a very large snack, verging on an out-of-control excessive amount of sweets. Simply stopping that was enough to trigger significant weight loss over time.

After a few more months, she was regaining weight, creeping back towards her previous weight. I didn't ask her about that, as I know it can be very distressing. But recently I see she's back to losing, having again given up sugar again.

It's easy to identify habits that keep the weight on. Changing those habits is hard. The All-Or-Nothing approach may not work for the long haul. You need to develop realistic coping strategies for the triggers and situations that contribute to bad eating habits.

Hunger

Here's one thing that drives me crazy about diets. The fear of hunger. Hunger is labeled The Enemy. We're told to snack and eat all the time and add this or that to meals to squelch hunger. As if one hunger pang will defeat all your good intentions. I'm here to say that true hunger – grumbling stomach and hunger pangs – is actually a good thing in the short term.

First, most of what fad diets label "hunger" is more likely to be psychological craving for something to eat, not actual physical metabolic *hunger*. It's more correctly described as appetite – the *desire* to eat food. When I ask obese people if they've felt hunger pangs, they look at me like I'm from outer space. They don't experience physiological hunger. Why? Because they're always eating, typically in response to appetite. They eat because they're bored, because it's the time of day to eat, because food is there in front of them, and so forth. Unfortunately, there are plenty of reasons to eat when you're not physically hungry.

When you haven't eaten for 4-5, or more, hours, your stomach empties out. Hormones start signaling that food is needed. In response, the muscles of your digestive system start contracting, creating something called the Migrating Motor Complex or MMC. According to the National Library of Medicine, the MMC is a housekeeping process, that flushes residues of digestion and any GI microbes hanging around out of the upper digestive system, to get ready for the next meal.

If you're always eating – meals, snacks, beverages, more snacks, another meal, etc. – the MMC never happens. You're always in a state of being fed. There's no cleansing housekeeping muscle contractions.

You probably remember when mothers said "no you can't have a cookie, it will ruin your appetite for dinner". Who does that anymore? Life is now about constant snacking. I'm here to say those mothers knew best. You should allow yourself to get hungry. You should eat a reasonable meal, go about your business, and 4 or so hours later eat another meal because you're hungry again. It's the way people used to eat, back when food had to be cooked from scratch and everyone had to wait for the meal to be served by the designated cook.

But won't all this hunger make you overeat at meals? Not necessarily. You might be surprised to find that less food fills you up faster when you're actually hungry. Of course, the key is to eat healthful food when you're hungry, not just stuff yourself with junk.

This is not a weight loss diet book, so I'm not going to on and on about this. Let me sum up the key points:

1. A primarily plant-based diet is the best choice because it's nutritious and fills you up. Many cuisines fit that description, from Mediterranean to Indian to Asian.
2. Make sure your meals have adequate protein, which also helps stifle appetite

3. Unless you have some unusual medical problem, low fat is not a good choice. Use healthy fats in moderate amounts to increase satiety.
4. Limit foods with added sugar. Especially soft drinks and sweets.
5. Limit alcohol.
6. Stick to 3 meals a day as much as possible. Constant snacking isn't a great plan. Experience between-meal hunger (NOTE: diabetics should consult with a registered dietitian about an appropriate meal/snack schedule).
7. Try to divide your food intake equally between meals as much as possible. Or at the very least, don't load most of your day's food intake in the evening.
8. Don't stress about counting calories. The more important strategy is to identify the source of unnecessary excess calories.
9. Exercise!

Quick Takes on Popular Fad Diets

Fad diets are the worst. They're typically divorced from normal foods and normal eating patterns, full of bizarre restrictions based on fear mongering and faux science. A fad diet teaches you nothing about how to eat. The diet is seen as temporary, as if it's going to fix your weight problem and then you can go back to your old habits, the ones that made you obese in the first place.

I've written a lot about different fad diets over the past 10 years on my blog Radio Nutrition. It's amazing how the same old diet ideas come back, re-packaged with a shiny new name and a new author. Here are a few examples of the latest fads:

Low Carb: What used to be called The Stillman Diet (low carb) morphed into Atkins which has morphed into variants like Dukan, South Beach or Paleo. The premise is that carbs are bad because they somehow cause weight gain. Never mind that in numerous countries around the globe, people are thin despite eating high carb diets.

One thing low carb diets do that some people find helpful is they severely restrict your food choices. No more ice cream or cupcakes or donuts or chips or bread or pizza or toast or bagels or pasta. Etc. So all the foods that tempt you to overeat are prohibited. What's left? Vegetables and meat, perhaps some cheese or yogurt and fruit. So you automatically stop overeating calories. You may lose weight, assuming the restrictions lead to lower calorie intake.

The problem is you can't keep this up for too long. You drift back to your old habits; you've learned nothing about how to eat a normal balanced diet; pretty soon you're regaining weight.

Intermittent Fasting: this idea has been around for a few years, promoted by a self-styled diet guru. There are variations on this theme, but basically you eat "normally" for 5 days a week and eat almost nothing on the two other days. People do report weight loss. The problem is we don't hear from the people who didn't lose weight, who overate on the 5 "normal" days and/or perhaps cheated a bit on the 2 fast days.

I'm not sure intermittent fasting is all that revolutionary. People have been eating more or less from day to day for thousands of years. Sometimes you eat little for a day or two if you're sick or stressed or anxious or even traveling. Your body can cope. You may even lose a little weight as a result, assuming you don't over-compensate when you're back to normal.

The Intermittent Fasting advocates claims this system resets metabolism. It may. There is ongoing research. I don't discount it, but you need to be eating a healthy balanced diet on the normal food days, not gorge on junk.

Ketogenic: this *extremely high fat* diet has been used for 100+ years to suppress seizures, especially in children prone to that problem. No one really understands why it works for that purpose. One (undesirable) side effect for these children is weight loss, so someone got the idea to promote ketogenic diets for weight loss.

The diet is extremely restrictive. I can't emphasize that enough. You must eat a diet that's 70% fat, with normal protein and almost no carbohydrates. Your meals will be dominated by butter, cream, oil, avocados, eggs, fatty cheeses, fatty meats and very small portions of nuts or nut butter (they have carbs and must be limited). You're allowed small amounts of leafy greens or mushrooms or other very low carb vegetables.

This can get really boring. It's also inherently unbalanced. All kinds of nutrients will be lacking. You can't stick with this for long, at which point transitioning back to a normal diet becomes problematic. You re-gain some weight when glycogen stores are rebuilt, because glycogen is stored in association with water. That can be disheartening. And again, following an extremely restrictive diet for awhile teaches you nothing about normal eating.

Low Fat: Low fat diets – 20% or less of calories as fat -- were all the rage for a few years back in the late 20th century. They've fallen out of favor, but we're left with the residual effects in grocery stores: low fat cheese, low fat ice cream, low fat milk, low fat this and that, and a continuing obsession with lean cuts of meat.

As I said before, low fat looks good on paper: eat lower fat versions of normal foods, which have fewer calories, and the numbers should add up to weight loss. If that were true, the obesity epidemic would have disappeared 20 years ago. In fact it's just gotten worse, and some people go so far as to blame low fat diets. People loaded up on low fat cookies and chips, thinking they had carte blanche to eat. They just ended up overeating carbohydrate calories.

But the main problem with low fat is that no one can stick to this type of diet for long. Low fat is just not satisfying. Research shows people drift back to their usual fat intake. Nevertheless, advocates continue to push low fat, and many people still buy low fat products. It's not inherently unhealthy; it's just not realistic for most people. If you do want to follow a low fat diet, you need to eat whole foods, not just a bunch of low fat processed foods.

Regaining

For plenty of people, the idea that you might find yourself in a situation where you need to *regain* weight is too outlandish to believe. Almost a dream come true – Woo hoo! 10 or 15 lbs just disappears! But unintended weight loss is usually associated with a medical problem or general effects of aging. Up to 20% of older adults are impacted. There are many potential causes for this type of weight loss:

- Illness that causes weight loss/loss of appetite, such as stroke, cancer or infection
- Medication that impacts taste or appetite
- Recovery from surgery or injury
- Malabsorption problems
- Swallowing or chewing problems
- Stress, depression or dementia leading to loss of appetite
- Unexplained reasons

Medical diagnosis of unintentional weight loss is defined as loss of more than 5% of body weight in 6-12 months. If you've previously been overweight, you might think at first "oh good, I've lost 5 pounds (or more) without even trying." Then it's 5 or 10 more pounds. As weight loss continues, you lose energy, fitness and stamina. Plenty of people would worry about that amount of unexplained weight loss, since it can be a sign of an underlying disease process. But many times metabolic and hormonal changes associated with aging are the cause.

Hormones that affect the digestive tract and hunger signals from the gut and brain change with age. Your stomach takes longer to empty, reducing appetite. You might feel full sooner due to other hormonal changes. Your senses of smell and taste may be reduced, so food seems less appetizing. Lack of physical activity, especially when you are sidelined by illness or injury can also impact appetite. And living alone, social isolation and resulting depression and apathy can impact food intake and food choices.

Unintentional weight loss can take on a life of its own. If you've been losing weight for any of the above reasons, you will have been under-consuming nutrients like protein, vitamins and minerals. Nutrient deficiencies can exacerbate malabsorption and further reduce appetite. This process can spiral out of control before you realize what happened.

According to the American Academy of Family Physicians, this type of weight loss is associated with increased risk for disease. This isn't surprising. You are losing muscle mass as well as fat, which will impact strength and energy. Eventually all organ systems are adversely impacted. Digestion becomes less efficient, and you absorb less of what you do eat. You can become more frail, and cognition and brain function can be negatively impacted. It's a vicious cycle, as many nutrient deficiencies contribute to further appetite suppression, depression and digestive disturbances.

In the absence of a serious unresolved medical situation, boosting nutrient intake and regaining some weight, or at least halting weight loss, is possible. But you have to be vigilant and you may have to eat even if you don't have any appetite. I've heard a colleague describe this as eating for the nutrition, not eating for pleasure. Food is now medicine that you must consume, preferably on a set schedule. It can seem like a chore.

You might think a weight gain diet includes all those treats you usually limit, like ice cream, French fries, donuts, cookies, pie, cakes and candy. Not so. While those might have some place in your diet, the bulk of your food should be nutrient dense with significant protein. You should plan to eat three meals a day, even if they are small to start with. Sticking to a schedule helps to keep you on track with consistent food intake.

To encourage healthy weight re-gain, add one or two snacks between meals. Beverages can be easier to consume and less filling, so one easy way to accomplish this is to use a nutrition supplement beverage. They come ready-to-drink in single-serve cans (Ensure, Boost, Nesquik, etc.) and powders (Carnation Instant Breakfast, for example). Or you or a family member can make smoothies with juice, milk or yogurt, a little protein powder and fresh fruit. Products marketed to muscle-building athletes would not be appropriate, as the ingredient mix will be different.

Commercial supplement beverages typically have about 300 calories per serving, with added vitamins, minerals and protein. Most are based on milk, although some are juice- or soy-based. You can mix the powdered varieties with soy milk if you prefer. Mixing with a plant milk results in drastically lower protein content, not advisable in this situation.

Basically the commercial supplement drinks are like flavored milk mixed with added vitamins and minerals. Some have extra protein, fiber or other specialized ingredients. Commercial drinks are more a matter of convenience. You can create your own between-meal snacks with everyday foods. The best snacks would be calorie-dense. While fresh vegetables and fruit are certainly healthy, they are also filling, so best to stick to higher calorie foods for a snack if you're trying to regain weight. Here are some examples:

- a PB & J with a small glass of milk
- a cup of yogurt (more protein in Greek style)
- toast with melted cheese
- cream soup made with milk
- smoothie made with juice, yogurt/milk, fresh fruit and a bit of sweetener if necessary
- tuna salad and half bagel

You probably can come up with your own ideas. Remember, the snack should have some significant amount of protein, which is important for regaining muscle. Even a donut and glass of milk is better than nibbling on candy and drinking sweetened tea.

Once you've halted the weight loss, and perhaps regained some weight, you still need to pay attention to your diet and your weight to avoid a repeat. Including high protein foods at all meals (see Chapter 6) will be especially important, as you don't want your regained weight to just be body fat. Stick to nutrient dense foods, like vegetables, fruits and whole grains. If fresh raw vegetables make you feel too full and cut your appetite, use cooked vegetables dishes more often.

Leave room in your diet for some treats and indulgences, but don't allow yourself to slip into an eating pattern that is primarily grab-'n-go processed food. You might prefer sweet flavors, but don't let your taste buds pull you away from healthy food.

Finally, it's very important to include regular physical activity to help stimulate digestion and appetite, and to build and maintain muscle. You are *never too old* to repair and rebuild muscle. *Never.* While you might not get back to the fitness level or muscle mass you had 15 or 20 years ago, you can still improve strength, stamina and mobility, and avoid debilitating frailty.

After significant weight loss, some people find it helpful to work with a trainer who understands the muscle building process for older adults. A physical therapist can also provide guidance on what muscle groups need attention. And don't underestimate less strenuous activities like walking. You don't need to do spin classes or military-style exercise classes to improve muscle strength. You do need to be persistent.

Eating disorders

Anorexia isn't just for teenagers anymore. Actually it never was, but the popular image is a teen girl starving herself to stick-thinness. In fact there are plenty of older women who have eating disorders, particularly restrictive eating leading to very low body weight.

Severe anorexia has a high mortality rate. Adolescents and young adults who do not recover may not survive to middle age. But thanks to modern medicine, many people with eating disorders lead long lives. They may struggle with recurrence of restrictive eating behavior over the years, triggered by life events. They may have developed coping strategies for those situations, such as a network of trusted family or friends to help them recover.

Anorexia can start at any age, and 50's, 60's and 70's are no exception. Medical problems that cause unintended weight loss are more common as we age. Illness or injury that disrupts food intake and leads to wasting can turn into anorexia. The person is happy with the weight loss and decides more weight loss is a good idea. Food intake is restricted even after the medical problem is resolved. While this might not lead to the skeletal frame of an anorexic, it's still disordered eating: deliberately restricting food intake to maintain an unnaturally thin body.

What could be wrong with that if you were previously overweight? If the food restriction leads to inadequate nutrient intake, new medical problems can result. As noted previously, poor protein intake contributes to muscle wasting and sarcopenia. Resulting frailty increases risk for numerous diseases. Poor intake of calcium and other bone-building minerals can compromise bone integrity, leading to osteoporosis and increased fracture risk and disability. Cognitive decline is linked to poor intake of many nutrients.

While there are many effective treatment options, there is a catch when it comes to adults. Parents of minor children are legally obligated to make treatment decisions for their children. An adult must make her own decision. No one else has legal responsibility. Adults cannot be forced into treatment. Since no one else is legally responsible, all the motivation has to originate with the person who has the eating disorder. Certainly that person can solicit help, but she is also free to ignore it.

Some eating disorder treatment centers now accept older adult patients. These centers have very effective programs, but they are also very disruptive to daily life. Inpatient treatment may take weeks, during which time you are away from your home and family and usual activities. Costs can be prohibitive, so while this type of intervention may be effective, it's not realistic for many people.

The basic message is this: there are older adults living with eating disorders. Regardless of how the eating disorder started, they put their health at risk. Older women should be eating an especially healthy diet, not compounding the effects of aging by restricting food choices.

A person in this situation needs to recruit a group of friends or family who will monitor her food intake and provide emotional support. Counseling with a psychotherapist who is experienced working with eating disordered clients is also advised. Anorexia in particular is not just a problem of eating too little. There are underlying psychological issues that need to be addressed to facilitate recovery and improved health.

Why?

You might be wondering what would lead an older woman to obsess about weight in such an extreme manner? Surely she doesn't aspire to look like an emaciated fashion model! The popular explanation for eating disorders is the influence of fashion magazines: images of thin women drive other women to obsess about weight, leading to binge eating or bulimia or anorexia. But how to explain why boys and men develop the same eating disorders? Or older women?

Theories abound. Most experts agree that eating disorders have a very strong genetic link, and that family life and peer pressure can push someone into the behavior. We think of binge eating as a form of self-medication, to boost feel-good brain chemicals. Another theory suggests *not* eating (anorexia) is a variation on self-medication, controlling brain signals in a different manner.

Eating disorders are not new to modern society. They've been documented for hundreds of years, long before fashion magazines. Fasting has an even longer history as an accepted part of religious life, supposedly leading to clarity of mind. Based on the appearance of some religious and cult figures, religious fasting looks pretty similar to anorexia, with a more culturally acceptable rationale.

The problem with eating disorders at older ages is not the thinner body; older adults can certainly be thin and healthy. The worry is the *extreme* food restricting behaviors or binge eating or bulimia, all of which lead to health problems that can severely impact an older woman's general health at a time of life when she needs to be eating the best possible diet.

15 CHRONIC DISEASES

I don't want to write a book about diseases, mainly because information about diet and chronic diseases is widely available from other reliable sources. No need to reinvent the wheel.

The common age-related chronic diseases linked to diet and lifestyle are:

1. Heart disease
2. Hypertension
3. Type 2 diabetes
4. Cancer
5. Osteoporosis
6. Arthritis
7. Cognitive impairment
8. Metabolic syndrome/inflammation

All these diseases and syndromes are linked to the same lifestyle factors: obesity, poor diet, sedentary lifestyle. Smoking, alcoholism and drug abuse are other detrimental factors. If you have Type 2 diabetes and you make a serious effort to reverse it with lifestyle changes, you also reduce your risk for heart disease, hypertension, cognitive impairment and possibly certain cancers.

I personally don't like to distinguish between these diseases for that reason. I don't like the way diet advice is dished out: "This diet will impact heart disease. This diet will impact Type 2 diabetes. This diet will impact hypertension." It's all the same diet – basically a Mediterranean style diet, or DASH diet, which is an Americanized version of Mediterranean.

Inflammation

Inflammation is your body's natural and proper reaction to injury or infection. Specialized cells and mediator molecules are mobilized to heal injuries, fight infective agents and protect the body from damage. We've all experienced localized inflammatory responses when, for example, we get a cut or bruise or contract a digestive or respiratory infection. Some conditions, such as arthritis, represent chronic inflammation.

The focus of so-called anti-inflammatory diets and foods is not the common localized types of inflammation that occur in response to an injury. Rather, it's the theoretical existence of a generalized and on-going whole body state of chronic inflammation. The problem is, there is no official diagnostic criteria for this generalized inflammation.

Nevertheless this is a hot topic and you can find hundreds or thousands of websites and books with advice on diets, foods and supplements that combat "inflammation". It's now popular to blame chronic inflammation for most of the chronic diseases listed above, along with plenty of other problems like digestive upset, skin problems, headaches and even obesity.

What are the facts? Who knows? Until we have really good research data (which would take years to collect and would need to be exhaustively detailed, making it an expensive and cumbersome undertaking), we don't have a good way to pin down a solid definition of chronic inflammation with measurable biomarkers and then link those to development of some disease process. It's entirely possible that the disease process and the inflammatory response are hard to distinguish as cause-and-effect. Heart disease might be caused by inflammation, or inflammation might be caused by heart disease.

So while I'm not jumping on the inflammation bandwagon, I do think it's very important, as we age, to maintain a lifestyle that supports our immune systems and normalizes inflammatory response, whether the response is to a paper cut on your finger or an allergen in the air. Support for specific anti-inflammatory foods or food components is not strong. Support for general diets and lifestyle factors is stronger, if only by association. The diet with the strongest link to immune function, along with reduced risk for chronic diseases is a plant-centric Mediterranean style diet.

What about anti-inflammatory foods?

When it comes to so-called anti-inflammatory foods, don't get me started. The amount of suggestive gobbledygook floating around is epic.

Here are some of my criticisms:
1. Lists of inflammatory (bad) or anti-inflammatory (good) foods with zero evidence to back up those lists. These lists are frequently reflections of the author's personal prejudices about foods. French fries and soft drinks are inflammatory? What's the evidence? That they aren't terribly healthful is a different matter entirely.
2. Conclusions about the health benefits of certain foods based on studies using isolated chemicals extracted from the food to treat isolated cells in a test tube. Suffice it to say, chemicals in food do not necessarily behave the same way once inside the body, interacting with live cells. Some of these wonder chemicals aren't even absorbed, or are quickly metabolized into something else, rendering them inactive.
3. Research on the wonderful benefits of a specific food that's funded by a trade group paid to promote that food.
4. Actual medical scientists who sling around advice on anti-inflammatory diets based on their own personal prejudices about foods. See #1 above.
5. Assuming that an effect on some biomarker actually translates into a measurable health benefit. While the levels of some molecule may go up or down in your blood, if that change doesn't impact your actual health, so what.

I suppose I shouldn't get so annoyed by this nonsense, since most of the advice points to the same sort of plant-centric diet I'd recommend anyway. Here's a summary list gleaned from a number of websites touting anti-inflammatory foods:

- Fatty fish (because of the omega-3 fat content)
- Whole grains
- Nuts (esp. almonds and walnuts)
- Olive oil
- Soy
- Coffee
- Sage
- Green tea
- Cayenne
- Cinnamon
- Beans
- Fruits and Veggies in general or specifically:
    - Peppers
    - Tomatoes
    - Leafy greens (kale, spinach)
    - Bok choy
    - Celery
    - Broccoli
    - Pineapple
    - Beets
    - Garlic/onions
    - Berries (esp blueberries)
    - Oranges
    - Avocadoes
    - Carrots
    - Tart cherries
- Flax seeds
- Chia seeds
- Coconut oil
- Ginger/turmeric
- Bone broth

The list of so-called pro-inflammatory foods reads like the

usual suspects: refined carbs, sugar, dairy, red meat. Evidence please?

Let's consider tart cherries, which are heavily promoted as an anti-inflammatory food. The evidence is mostly from research done on athletes, related to exercise performance and muscle recovery after exertion. Typically a small group of highly trained young athletes consume a tart cherry product, such as concentrated tart cherry powder, before exercising in a lab setting. Performance and recovery parameters are measured.

Consumption of tart cherry products is associated with some benefit in reducing soreness or enhancing endurance and recovery. Result: tart cherries show up on all the anti-inflammatory food lists. The powders are added to processed foods or supplements, to make the products look healthy. Unsurprisingly, many of these studies are funded by companies that grow tart cherries and/or produce and sell tart cherry extracts and powders.

Another Potential Cause

All the focus on alleged anti-inflammatory foods may be distracting us from one of the more important causes: obesity. Regardless of what specific foods you might eat, excess body fat can contribute to overall inflammation. Studies that compare body fat percentage – not weight – to inflammatory markers show this link.

How does this work? One expert explains it like this: as people gain fat weight and become obese, fat tissue expands and the fat cells enlarge. The blood supply to fat tissue can't keep up with cell needs. Cells die off, and as they die they release molecules that aggravate inflammation. Macrophages move in to clean up the dead cells. This process can happen regardless of body weight, in other words in a woman who is normal weight but high body fat.

The obesity connection to chronic inflammation is not solved by eating blueberries or almonds. The only solution for that is weight loss, particularly reduction of body fat.

Take Away

Am I opposed to the concept of the anti-inflammatory food list? I'm not opposed to the foods themselves (except... Coconut oil? Bone broth? Seriously?). In fact, it reads like a basic plant-based diet. If you're more inclined to adopt that type of diet because it's labeled "anti-inflammatory," so be it. If you're going to buy a food extract or powder or supplement, it's buyer beware. Don't expect miracles.

Continuing research is likely, as we understand more about the impact of diet and nutrition on inflammatory diseases like arthritis or lupus. Research on specific conditions like those might yield information that's useful for inflammation in general. Meanwhile we need a better way to measure what we call inflammation so we can better understand how to control it.

Cardiovascular Disease

We may all fear cancer, but heart disease is the #1 killer of older women. Recently, medical science has recognized that symptoms of this disease are very different between men and women, but different symptoms don't mean less severity.

Dietary advice on heart disease prevention has changed rather radically since we were children. Once the link between blood cholesterol and heart attacks was established, it was easy to leap to the conclusion that cholesterol in food caused heart attacks. Eggs were blamed, along with butter, cheese and shrimp. Margarine sales grew; egg consumption plummeted. Heart disease got worse.

Next we were told that saturated fat was the culprit, so butter was still on the hit list, along with red meat and whole milk. Low fat milk crowded out whole milk on store shelves. Foods like cheese and ice cream were re-engineered to reduce fat. Leaner cuts of meat were promoted. We got low fat versions of junky processed foods like cookies and chips. The American Heart Association and other public health agencies promoted low fat diets and effectively put the stamp of approval on all these low fat products. Heart disease didn't go away.

Recently, the heart disease diet saga veered into conspiracy theories, with claims that the research was rigged to blame fat and hide the fact that sugar is the true culprit. Adding to the argument, mounting evidence pointed to the higher fat Mediterranean style diet as the most effective strategy for reducing disease risk. A new set of diet gurus have now gone full circle and are promoting saturated fat – from coconut and butter – as healthful. Meanwhile the American Heart Association and US Dietary Guidelines have quietly liberalized fat and egg restrictions.

So where do we stand? Heart disease is a complicated multi-factorial disease. Lifestyle is a very significant piece of the puzzle, but so are genetics and environment. Lifestyle is the one thing you do have control over.

Calcium supplements and heart disease

Recent reports of a link between heart attack and calcium intake scared many women off supplements. Many studies have been done and findings are all over the map. For example, heart attack risk was associated with:

- total calcium intake
- supplemental calcium only for men
- low calcium intake
- high blood levels of calcium

Many studies found no association. Excessive intake from supplements is not advisable in any event. If you're taking calcium and are concerned about this, you should consult your physician.

Current Wisdom

As you can see from the history of diet advice above, current wisdom could easily change in the future. Still, the risk factors with the strongest link to increased risk include:

1. Sedentary lifestyle
2. High saturated fat intake
3. Poor intake of vegetables and fruit
4. High sodium, especially associated with a diet high in cured/processed meats, processed foods and fast foods
5. High sugar intake.

The diet most closely associated with reduced risk is the Mediterranean style diet. The DASH (Dietary Approaches to Stop Hypertension) Diet is closely related. Vegetarian and Flexitarian diets can also fit this description, as can many Asian cuisines. Whatever you call it, the main features are:

1. Plant-based: most of the foods in a meal or snack should be sourced from plant foods, including vegetables, fruit, legumes, nuts and whole grain food products.
2. A limit on sugary sweets, beverages and desserts. These types of foods may be eaten only occasionally.
3. Moderate fat intake, primarily from vegetable oils.
4. Small portions of fish, meats, poultry, eggs and dairy (depending on vegetarian preferences)
5. Daily physical activity

In addition to being heart healthy, this type of eating plan is packed with nutrients and fiber. Not to mention the possibilities for delicious creative recipes and flavors are endless. What's not to like? The old way of thinking about a heart healthy diet – based on tasteless low fat processed foods; feeling deprived of flavor – is over.

It's the Whole Diet

Nutrition for heart health is about the whole diet. It's not about taking some supplement or antioxidant or herb or loading up on an alleged 'super food'. None of those will fix a poor diet. Knowledge about heart healthy eating is expanding as new research results are published. We may know more in the future about the interaction of nutrients and genes that impact heart disease and blood pressure, leading to more personalized recommendations. At the moment, you can act to reduce your risks by way of your diet and exercise.

Here's a final tip: if you're obese/over-fat, reducing fat weight is another way to influence your risk for many chronic diseases, including heart disease, Type 2 diabetes, metabolic syndrome and several cancers. Happily, plant based diets are also associated with better weight control, but you still have to make healthful choices. Technically, sugar and vegetable oils are made from plants. A plant-based diet can be loaded with chips, pastries and French fries. Not exactly a recipe for health.

Hypertension

High blood pressure, or hypertension, is frequently included in the cardiovascular disease category. Elevated blood pressure is a risk factor for heart attack, but also for stroke. While many of the same lifestyle factors that impact heart disease risk are linked to blood pressure, there are some specific differences that can be impacted by diet.

While doctors will typically prescribe medication for blood pressure problems, diet changes are essential in most cases. Weight loss to the normal weight range can result in lower blood pressure.

One standard recommendation for hypertension is to

> ### Sodium in foods
>
> To their credit, some food manufacturers have quietly been reducing salt content of many popular products with no publicity. Why? Consumers believe that foods labeled "reduced sodium" won't taste good. So less salt is used without fanfare. This isn't a bad thing. Overall it means people who buy certain processed foods are in fact eating less salt without even noticing.

reduce salt (sodium) intake. There's been a lot of push-back on this concept recently, particularly from medical experts. Official recommendations in the US keep pinching the ideal sodium intake to extremely low levels. It now stands at 1500 mg/day, down from 2500 mg. This new restriction pretty much precludes eating anything prepared outside your own kitchen, even down to loaf bread and cheese. Meanwhile other experts argue that more liberal sodium intakes are well tolerated and these new recommendations are too extreme.

One problem with blanket recommendations for entire populations is genetics. Some people are so-called "salt sensitive" – their blood pressure reacts more to sodium than other peoples'. But who is salt sensitive? You'd have to pay for a genetic test to find out, and how many people are willing to do that?

The focus on salt has obscured some important diet issues. One is that potassium plays a very significant role in regulating blood pressure. And potassium is one mineral that is commonly under-consumed. It's especially concentrated in vegetables in fruits. Statistics show that most people eat few of these important foods. Worse, diets based on high salt processed foods exacerbate the problem. Potassium and sodium need to be balanced. Instead the average person consumes far more sodium than potassium.

This is one reason every health advocacy organization under the sun recommends eating generous portions of vegetables and fruit. Potassium must be consumed in its natural form; it can't be used to fortify food, and supplemental potassium is problematic. So instead of fortified processed foods with "high potassium!" labels, we get processed foods that are "reduced sodium" or "low sodium". They're still processed foods, but now they have a health halo. People think they're doing themselves a favor buying low sodium soup, while ignoring high potassium foods.

Type 2 Diabetes

Rates of this once-rare lifestyle disease have skyrocketed in the past 20-30 years. While Type 2 diabetes is a problem with blood sugar control, it is distinctly different from Type 1. In Type 2, your body still makes insulin, but your cells don't listen to it properly. Insulin signals cells to take up glucose. If the cells can't get the signal, blood glucose builds up to unhealthy levels (see Chapter 17 for more details about insulin and glucose). In Type 1 diabetes, the body does not make insulin, so it must be injected. In Type 2, medications can correct the glucose-clearing signaling system.

Type 2 diabetes is strongly related to obesity and a sedentary lifestyle. Simply losing weight goes a long way to reversing symptoms. If you have Type 2 diabetes, you should consult with a registered dietitian nutritionist, preferably one who specializes in diabetes. Your physician should be able to refer you to someone, preferably with the Certified Diabetes Educator credential. CDE indicates a person has the higher level of education and experience needed to work with diabetics. Since diabetes demands an exacting treatment and diet program, it's a very good idea to have professional guidance.

Don't take this lightly. Type 2 diabetes ups your risk for kidney disease and heart disease and is associated with certain cancers.

Cancer

Many common cancers are linked to obesity. Whether the obesity, or the obesity-causing lifestyle is the key is unclear. But major cancers like breast and colon cancer are on this list. For breast cancer, obesity is associated with increased risk for the cancer to recur after treatment, and for the recurrence to be more aggressive.

Studies of breast cancer patients suggest that weight loss as part of the initial treatment phase can help prevent those recurrences. Of course, this is dependent on initial weight, type of cancer and stage of disease. If you were diagnosed while at a normal weight, losing more weight is not likely to help.

Cancer itself and cancer treatments can lead to weight loss, sometimes dramatic weight loss. While this might sound like a good idea to overweight people, this type of weight loss is not healthy. It typically involves significant loss of muscle mass. Your strength and energy deteriorate, and recovery can be impaired. Depending on the type of cancer, your providers will likely have advice on maintaining weight and strength during treatment.

Cancer patients should consult with a dietitian who specializes in cancer nutrition and diets. Different cancers create different diet/nutrition issues. Additionally treatments can affect your ability to ingest and digest food, which can contribute to unhealthy weight loss and poor outcomes. Some medications interact with foods. A dietitian will anticipate those problems and help you work through them, to enhance treatment effects and recovery.

The Big Picture

Nutrition and diet have enormous impacts on risk for chronic diseases and on recovery from those diseases. Entire books have been written about the nutrition and lifestyle issues for any of these conditions. As this book is not focused so much on diseases, I didn't want to reinvent the wheel, so to speak.

These are the key Take Away points:

1. In general, the best diet for health is a plant-based diet, whether you call it Mediterranean or DASH or flexitarian or vegetarian or give it some other name. Research links this type of diet to reduced risk for cardiovascular disease, Type 2 diabetes, hypertension and many cancers.
2. People with cancer, Type 2 diabetes and less common chronic diseases (Parkinson's Disease is one example) should consult a Registered Dietitian Nutritionist for personalized guidance on the best diet plan for their situation. This is particularly true

for cancer patients, as different cancers and treatments call for specific dietary intervention.

3. Healthful weight loss to a normal weight range helps reduce risk factors. Added bonus of plant-centric diets: they're associated with lower body weight and easier weight control.

You can find plenty of resources on diets for chronic diseases online and from books. You can also find plenty of unreliable factoids, typically used to market supplements, foods and diet books. There is a list of the more reliable websites in the General References section at the end of the book.

THE NEXT SECTION PREVIEW
IT'S ALL ABOUT FOOD

Shocking! Somehow humans survived for hundreds of thousands of years with food as the only source of nutrients. Well, let's clarify that concept. Long ago, humans lived much shorter lives, they generally weren't very tall and they certainly were more physically active and thinner. They were also subject to nutritional deficiencies when food supply was scarce or unbalanced. So yes nutrition depended entirely on food, but it wasn't always optimal. Now, we think of nutrition as pills, powders and fortified processed foods.

Foods are being medicalized or demonized, frequently based more on rumor, myth and marketing ploys than actual facts. So-called super foods are alleged to cure diseases single-handedly. Food products are created to take advantage of nutrient buzzwords. Energy bars with a sprinkling of B-vitamins, fiber, omega-3 fats or some powdered super food extract are common examples. Individual foods or entire food groups are blamed for all our ills. Some foods swing back and forth between 'super-ness' and demonization, depending on the research-du-jour. Those stories may be good click-bait on the internet, but they don't make for a coherent diet plan.

The following chapters are about food, which after all is the whole point of eating. You'll find information about major food components, health claims both good and bad, explanations of where a food fits into a balanced diet, and examples of what that diet might look like for the average older and food-wiser woman.

16 HEALTH HALO FOODS

What's the scoop on health halo marketing terms like "super food" and "organic"? Hint: one is far more useful than the other for guiding food choices.

Super Foods

In my not-humble but decidedly professional opinion, the entire idea of super foods is ridiculous. No one food is going to save you from poor health, and no one food can cancel out the effects of an over-all junky diet. Where did this idea come from? It's a relatively recent phenomenon, fueled by producers and trade organizations that fund research to hunt for any potential health benefits of their food product. Any data showing any kind of benefit at all is used for promotional purposes. In many cases, very minor or inconsequential "benefits" are pumped up to look like a big deal to unsuspecting consumers.

Interestingly, most of the "super food" claims are for plant foods, particularly vegetables and fruits. In fact, it seems like every vegetable or fruit has been labeled a "super food" at one time. Raspberries, acai, blueberries, sour cherries and pomegranate are just some examples. Other plant foods, such as almonds, walnuts and, more recently, coconut are examples. Who can argue that any of those shouldn't be part of a balanced diet? They're not bad foods, but *super*?

Someone could write an exposé on the association between research funding entities and super-food claims. Published research studies may declare funding sources right in the study document, so if you have access to the original publication, you can usually find out who paid for a study. Or you can use my approach: when you see something promoted as a Super Food, the first word that pops into your mind is "marketing". If you like that particular food, fine. Just don't expect miracles.

Chocolate: The Super Food We Love to Love

Chocolate is another great example of the marketing power of research grants. We love chocolate for the rich flavor. But chocolate companies are betting on the marketing potential of health benefits, and have funded plenty of studies to look for evidence. Chocolate contains flavanols, a class of antioxidant, linked by some research to health benefits like improved blood vessel integrity, lower blood pressure or lower risk for Type 2 diabetes. So the evidence exists, but it's not monumental and it's not consistent. The marketing value makes it worthwhile, helping to sell all manner of cocoa-derived products, from cocoa powder capsules to dark chocolate bars.

There's nothing wrong with a little chocolate, especially if it satisfies your appetite for a treat and keeps you from scarfing down a half-gallon of ice cream. It might provide a minor health benefit, but it's not going to fix an otherwise junky diet.

If you're interested in pursuing the apparent health benefits of chocolate, one of the most effective ways to consume the suggested daily dose of 200 mg of flavanols is to eat ½ ounce of unsweetened baking chocolate. Too bitter and medicinal? If you're really looking for an excuse to eat chocolate, stick to dark chocolate. You aren't going to get any meaningful amount of flavanols from chocolate ice cream or chocolate brownies or chocolate chip cookies.

Organic

Back in the 1970's, Joni Mitchel sang:

"Give me spots on my apples
But leave me the birds and the bees...please!"

It was the early years of the organic food movement, a tiny niche market limited to the world of hippies and Back-to-the-

Earthers. Many of you remember those days and may have been early advocates for organic food. Now organic is mainstream. In the US, we've had national standards since 1990, so that organic in Vermont is the same as organic in Arizona. You can buy organic food at Walmart and your average grocery store. You can buy organic chips and soft drinks. Is this progress?

Organic food is grown without chemical pesticides, growth hormones, synthetic fertilizers or bioengineering. Organic farmers are expected to practice soil and water conservation and use of renewable resources. All of this is time-consuming, which explains why organic food is typically more expensive than conventionally produced foods. But some people believe the extra expense is worth it, if it means not consuming unknown pesticide residues.

There's a persistent belief that organic foods are more nutritious. Research comparing foods produced with organic vs. conventional techniques is inconclusive. Sometimes the food looks more nutritious; sometimes it looks no different. The problem is how the comparisons are done. For example, the biggest influence on produce nutrient content is soil, along with weather conditions during the growing season. Comparing tomatoes from an organic farm to tomatoes grown on a distant conventional farm under different conditions is not exactly fair. Another problem is seed variety. Mass-produced tomatoes may all be one hybrid type, which may not look nutritionally equivalent to an heirloom tomato grown on organic soil. So it's hard to make a blanket conclusion one way or another. For most people, flavor is the overriding factor. If a locally grown organic tomato tastes fabulous compared to a so-so tennis-ball tomato at the grocery store, and you don't mind paying $6 for a tomato, you'll buy the organic one.

The term "organic" was originally associated with produce, such as Joni Mitchell's wormy apples. Not anymore. Organic is everywhere, from the dairy case to the meat counter to the chip aisle. Food manufacturers are always looking for a marketing advantage. Organic food is mainstream; "organic" is used as a health halo marketing gimmick You can find organic chips, soft drinks, cookies, ice cream and sugary breakfast cereals. Does organic make these things healthier? Does organic make them worth more money? I trust you know the answer to those questions.

Local food frequently factors into the organic decision-making process, especially at farmer's markets. Local and organic are not equivalent terms, although many local growers use organic techniques. But many large scale farms hundreds of miles away produce certified organic food. Again, price and flavor may be the deciding factors.

Keep in mind, neither organic nor local guarantees safety. A food may be grown without pesticides, but that doesn't mean it can't be contaminated with dangerous bacteria. Listeria, salmonella and e. coli do not care that your tomato or melon or eggs were grown organically. Producers and consumers still have to practice safe food handling, including washing and storage.

The words "Clean" and "Natural" sound shiny and healthy when applied to food or diets. Who wants to eat food that's dirty or unnatural? In truth, these are meaningless terms. Unlike "organic", there is no official regulated definition of either clean or natural.

So is it a problem if you don't buy organic foods? Are you more likely to develop dire diseases? We've been eating foods grown with synthetic fertilizers and treated with pesticides for many years. There's no clear evidence that particular diseases are caused by any of that. Safety studies done on rodents fed enormous amounts of a pesticide may find an increase in cancer, but how meaningful is that for a human who is exposed to minute doses? People who stick to organic food may claim they are healthier, but they are also likely to be following other healthy lifestyle practices. At the moment there are no definitive answers.

Pesticide residues aside, one benefit of organic food production is better soil management, less fertilizer run off polluting water supplies and alternative livestock management practices. The demand for organic food encourages experimentation and research into better farming practices. Buying organic food supports this new system, which increases interest among other farmers and food manufacturers. So to that end, organic food is a good thing. Back in the 1970's, buying organic apples with worms was a badge of honor. Now, thanks to enormous progress in organic farming techniques, organic apples look as unblemished as conventionally grown apples.

17 SHOULD YOU FEAR CARBOHYDRATES?

It's very popular to blame all our ills on carbohydrates. Sugar, white flour, anything made with white flour, gluten (also white flour), white foods in general, potatoes and even milk (it contains the sugar lactose) are the components of thousands of food products that people enjoy. They're frequently high calorie and low nutrient, making them easy targets for the carb-phobes.

Carbohydrates in food (sugars and starches) are made up of sugar molecules linked together. Starches are long chains of sugars; sugars may be single molecules (such as glucose or fructose) or double (glucose + fructose, which is sucrose). Whatever the form, carbohydrates are broken down into the individual sugar units during digestion, and then absorbed into the blood.

> I sometimes wonder about the cultural basis for this anti-carb hysteria. Common carbohydrate foods are inexpensive and widely available. Meanwhile diets like Paleo, Atkins and other meat-heavy regimens are expensive. Is it an elitist/class thing? Many of the so-called super foods are expensive, too. Five dollars for a tiny tray of fresh raspberries? It does make me wonder about the origins of carb phobia.

Glucose is the primary sugar in blood and the primary energy source for cells. It's guided into cells by the hormone insulin. Sugars in excess of short term energy needs are stored for future use as glycogen (a storage form of carbohydrate) or fat. Insulin levels increase as blood glucose increases, and then drop off as glucose levels decrease.

That's the short and simple description of how your body handles the carbohydrates you eat. Here's how the carbphobes would explain it:

*When you eat those awful carbs, your blood sugar SPIKES!!! Insulin **pours** into your system, and your blood sugar CRASHES!!! You feel shaky. You become comatose. You get diabetes! And heart disease!! Carbs are TOXIC!!!*

It's a wonder anyone is left alive. At the very least, the streets should be littered with the bodies of people who ate a bagel or a croissant for breakfast.

Keep in mind, this glucose control system has been operational for eons. It's normal for blood sugar to increase after eating. And it's normal for insulin to be released to move that glucose into cells, at which point blood glucose levels go down. *That's how it works.* Describing it as some kind of pathological problem is false.

Humans have eaten carbohydrate-heavy diets for millennia. Paleo advocates aside, most of the calories consumed by hunter-gatherer societies were carbohydrates from roots, seeds, leaves, fruits and tubers. Cultivation of grains like wheat and rice also contributed carbs to the diet. Many cultures today still rely on high carbohydrate diets, especially in the developing world.

High carbohydrate foods can be divided into two general categories:

1. Unrefined: whole grains and foods made with whole grains, fruits, vegetables, legumes, nuts.
2. Refined: sugar and sweeteners, white rice, white flour and foods made with white flour (bread, pasta, hamburger buns, pizza crust, donuts, cookies, etc.)

Unfortunately, refined carbohydrate foods seem to have taken over much of the food supply in developed countries. Why? Many of these foods are nutritionally sketchy, at best. But then few people pick foods solely on the basis of nutrition. Taste, convenience and cost are the main deciding factors. And these types of foods taste good. Plus they're convenient, they keep well and they're generally inexpensive.

The list of foods in that second category seems endless: soft drinks, cereals, white bread, pasta, pastries, cookies, chips, snack foods like pretzels, cakes, candy, frozen desserts like ice cream. Truthfully you could do fine with a diet that excluded all of these. For most people that's just not realistic. It also might not be that beneficial, considering that several of these foods are staples in countries where the population is generally (1) thinner and (2) healthier, such as France (bread), Italy (pasta) and Asian countries (white rice).

Carbohydrate foods are essential parts of a balanced diet, preferably in whole unprocessed unrefined forms. The problem is *which* carbohydrate foods make up the bulk of your food choices? The preferred choices are whole or relatively unprocessed varieties, low in added sugars and salt.

When your diet includes lots of sugary and refined carb foods, your insulin-release system has to work overtime and can become less effective. When insulin can't communicate with cells as effectively, blood glucose remains elevated. The medical term is insulin resistance, and it's a key feature of Type 2 diabetes. One key intervention for Type 2 diabetes is to control the carbohydrate content of meals to control blood glucose levels.

Easy to Overeat

Here's another problem with a diet that's heavy on refined carbohydrate foods: calories. It's extremely easy to overeat these foods. They're tasty, they're frequently high fat and high calorie, and they're not filling. You can fit a lot of potato chips or ice cream in your stomach before you notice you're full. Chronic over-consumption of calories leads to weight gain, which in itself increases Type 2 diabetes, heart disease, hypertension and other diseases.

It's hard to over-eat calories of whole unrefined carb foods like vegetables, whole grains, legumes and fruit. Plus they are not digested and absorbed as quickly because the fiber in these foods slows the process down. In any event, we don't typically just eat one food. We eat mixed meals or snacks. The speed of digestion and absorption will depend not just on the type of carbohydrate you eat. It depends on the fat, protein and fiber content of the meal, as well as fluid intake and total amount of food.

Take Away Message on Carbs
1. No they're not universally bad or toxic.
2. Yes you should limit consumption of sugary foods.
3. No you should not be fearful of carbohydrates in general.

18 IS FAT PHOBIA REASONABLE?

Fats have a reputation as both healthy and unhealthy. We've been told to avoid the saturated fat in butter, cheese and beef while loading up on olive oil and other vegetable oils. Coconut oil is now touted as a health food. Margarine has been re-engineered to remove trans fats, which are considered to be unhealthy.

One of the problems with talking about "fats" is that there the fats in our food come in different shapes and sizes, which are channeled into different metabolic pathways depending on those shapes and sizes. Fats can be:

- Stored in fat cells for future energy use
- Incorporated into structures like cell walls
- Metabolized into hormones and other molecular mediators
- Burned for fuel

Fats are basically long chains of carbon units attached to hydrogen atoms. Their shapes depend on how long the chains are (anywhere from 2 to 24 carbons long), whether any of those carbons are attached by a double bond rather than a single bond, how many double bonds there are and where on the chain the first double bond occurs. Complicated enough? This is simplified somewhat by the fact that double bonds are only found in chains of 18 or more carbon units.

Another complication: foods rarely contain just one type of fat. Most are mixtures of a variety of fatty acids. For example, the USDA food composition database, whole milk contains at least 12 different fatty acids, most of them saturated. Olive oil lists more than 10, most of which are monounsaturated.

To further complicate the issue, fatty acids in food are typically in triglyceride form. This is a 3-carbon backbone (glycerol) with a fatty acid attached to each of the 3 carbons. Hence the "tri" glyceride name. Sort of like a strange short comb with 3 very long teeth, although the teeth can be different lengths and some will have bends. During digestion, the fatty acids are detached from the glycerol before absorption. Triglycerides may be reformed elsewhere in the body. This is the storage form of fats in fat cells.

You don't need to understand the chemistry, just that the type of bond and the location of the bond on the carbon chain determines the shape. And shape determines function.

Saturated Fats

Chemically speaking, saturation means no double bonds in the carbon chain. All of the carbon-to-carbon links are single bonds, making the fat molecule rather straight, as molecules go. Double bonds, by contrast, create kinks and bends in the chain.

These fats come in many different lengths. You may have heard of medium chain triglycerides, which refers to fatty acids that are 6-12 carbons in length. Short chain means less than 6, and long chain is 14 or more.

Saturated fat intake is linked to increased risk for heart disease. A high intake usually increases LDL cholesterol. Cutting back on saturated fat intake is one recommendation for lowering LDL. Most of the research never distinguished between the different lengths of saturated fats that predominate in certain foods.

Now we have push back, with claims that high saturated fat foods like coconut are healthy (or at least not unhealthy) because they have a different mix of saturated fats compared to beef. This controversy isn't going away anytime soon. You'll likely continue to hear arguments for both sides in the debate. Meanwhile the official American Heart Association recommendation is to limit saturated fat intake to 5-6% of daily calories. That's about 9-10 grams/day for a woman eating about 1500 calories. The US Dietary Guidelines have a slightly more generous limit of 17 grams or less.

How do you know how much saturated fat you eat? You won't know unless you meticulously track your daily food intake with one of the many web-based food trackers. Or you can simply limit intake of high saturated fat foods:

- Butter
- Cream
- Cheese
- Red meat
- Poultry skin
- Coconut oil

So what about coconut oil? Yes it's highly saturated. And yes the fatty acids are primarily medium chain, which are metabolized differently. There's some evidence that eating a lot of this will raise LDL cholesterol, so the official recommendation is to limit intake. Other people argue that medium chain fats are actually healthy, going so far as to advocate switching to coconut fat entirely. Until there is definitive research, requiring time and money, this argument isn't going away anytime soon. Meanwhile unless you deliberately buy coconut fat to use for cooking, your exposure to it will be minimal.

Monounsaturated Fats

Monounsaturated fatty acids (MUFA) have one double bond in the carbon fatty acid chain, hence the prefix "mono". That double bond gives the chain one slight bend. MUFA intake is associated with lower LDL cholesterol and less risk for heart disease and insulin resistance.

MUFAs tend to solidify at cold temperatures. That's why olive oil – 73% MUFA – that's kept in the fridge will solidify. In fact olive oil is famous for its monounsaturated fat content, which is thought to account for many of the health benefits of a Mediterranean diet. But other foods have significant monounsaturated fat content:

- Avocado
- Nuts and nut butters

- Canola oil
- Beef fat, lard and lamb fat

Yes the fats in red meat have significant MUFAs, along with the saturated fat, illustrating the point that food fats are rarely just one type of fatty acid.

So should you eat more high MUFA foods? Many of the high MUFA foods listed above are part of a plant-centric diet. Using olive or canola oil for cooking and salad dressings and adding avocado, nuts and nut butters to meals and snacks is a good way to accomplish this goal. Adding more lard or high fat beef isn't the best plan. You'd have to eat a lot more calories from those to get the MUFA content of a couple of teaspoons of olive oil. So while you'll get some monounsaturates when you eat high fat red meats, you're better off focusing on the plant sources.

Polyunsaturated Fats

"Poly" unsaturated fatty acid (PUFA) chains have more than one double bond. You may have heard the term omega-6, and you read about omega-3 fatty acids in previous chapters. The "omega" refers to the location of the first double bond on the carbon chain. It's at the 6th carbon in omega-6 fats and the 3rd carbon on omega-3 chains. The shape of a PUFA is determined by the location of that first double bond and by the number of double bonds along the chain.

Have you ever opened a bottle of vegetable oil and realized it was rancid? That's because double bonds between carbon atoms are fragile, and prone to reacting with oxygen. This is undesirable in a food fat. It's called oxidation and it's a common problem for vegetable oils that are kept for long periods, especially in a warm environment or in sunlight. Saturated fats aren't prone to this problem, because they don't have double bonds.

Oxidized fatty acids are not nutritionally useful, because their shape and chemical reactivity have been altered. Oxidized oils should be discarded. Foods that contain oils can also become rancid. Examples include snack foods like chips and crackers, nuts, nut butters and oil-based salad dressings.

Fish oil, whether in capsules or liquid form, can also go rancid, which is why refrigerated storage is recommended.

PUFAs have a health halo. When people switch from a diet high in saturated fats to one with more vegetable oils, cholesterol levels decrease. For this reason, vegetable oils are recommended in heart healthy diets. But recently that health halo has gone askew. The saturated fat promoters claim that PUFAs, particularly the ubiquitous omega-6 variety, are pro-inflammatory and are therefore unhealthy. What is the basis of their claim?

Inflammation is a complex process, controlled by numerous signaling molecules, cells and metabolic systems. Some inflammatory mediators are made from long chain fatty acids. In general, mediators made from omega-6 fats can create an excessive inflammatory response when compared to mediators made from omega-3 fats. Remember, the double bonds in those fatty acid chains determine the shape and function. Omega-3 fats have a different shape than omega-6.

This has given rise to a popular new theory that claims chronic inflammation is caused by the high level of omega-6 fats in our food. According to this theory, cutting back on vegetable oils, particularly PUFA-rich oils, is healthier because it reduces inflammation. Conclusion: eat more saturated fat which doesn't impact inflammatory mediators.

So what's the truth here? As I noted in the section on inflammation, the jury is out on exactly how chronic inflammation is measured, and what type of diet is best for reducing it. A Mediterranean style diet has a good track record when it comes to diseases that involve inflammation. This diet emphasizes olive oil, which is high in monounsaturated fats, which are not metabolized to inflammatory mediators.

Evidence aside, what do *I* think of this theory? In my professional opinion, I think it has merit. I don't think a diet that's heavy on vegetable oils (other than olive oil) is a great plan. What would such a high omega-6 diet look like?

- You cook with oils or soft margarines or spreads.
- You put those types of spreads on toast and sandwiches.

- You use a lot of mayonnaise and salad dressing.
- You eat lots of foods made with vegetable oils: chips, crackers, bakery items and other processed foods including commercially prepared sauces or gravies
- You eat lots of commercially deep fried foods like French fries or fried chicken, or foods cooked on a griddle like pancakes, eggs, vegetables and burgers.

This might sound extreme, but in fact this describes how plenty of people eat day to day. Thanks to the decades-old mantra to eat less saturated fat, people are eating a lot more vegetable fats. Food intake studies support this statement. Consequently we now consume a larger portion of fats as omega-6 fatty acids compared to decades ago. Omega-6 fatty acids are metabolized to inflammatory mediators, some of which can intensify inflammatory responses, compared to the mediators made from omega-3 fats.

The scenario makes intuitive nutritional sense, and there's some evidence to back it up, but it's not conclusive. Should you dump your vegetable oils down the drain and switch to butter? I don't advise that. I don't advise eating excessive amounts of *any* fat for another very good reason. Fat is high calorie. Consider this: a teaspoon of a fat – oil, butter – has about 40 calories. A teaspoon of sugar has 16. You can fit a lot of fat calories in your stomach before you notice. Only a small amount of the fat you eat is metabolized to hormones, signal molecules and cell structures. The rest is burned for fuel or stored in fat cells. And when it comes to storing excess fat, your body doesn't care if it's saturated, mono or poly unsaturated. It's fat. It's stored. There is no way to flush excess fat out.

The best advice is summed up with unexciting term "moderation". A plant-based diet will contain a mix of fats by default. If you use olive oil, you'll have a considerable intake of monounsaturates. If you include small amounts of meats and cheese, you have some intake of saturated fat. If you use butter or cream, those also have more saturated fat. You might use foods made with vegetable oils sometimes. In general, if your diet is based on whole foods rather than processed foods, you'll have much more control over which fats are in your diet.

Trans Fats

Decades ago, when saturated fats were blamed for heart disease, margarine was promoted as the go-to butter substitute. Margarine and its cousin vegetable shortening are made with vegetable oils. But oils are liquid at room temperature and when refrigerated. What to do? Hydrogenation to the rescue.

The hydrogenation process reacts hydrogen with those double bonds in the PUFA-rich vegetable oils, making the fatty acids behave more like saturated fat, even though a chemically altered double bond remains. There's a catch. When the double bonds in PUFAs are altered this way, the resulting fatty acid does not have a natural shape. Instead of the natural bend of a PUFA or the straight line of a saturated fat, these trans fats have a kink (The term "trans" refers to the fact that hydrogen atoms at this double bond location are on opposite sides of the molecule, instead of on the same side, as found in naturally occurring molecules).

For years this process was seen as a great thing, a way to have your butter and eat it too, so to speak. Then health researchers realized that high intake of these trans fats was linked to elevated cholesterol and heart disease. It became increasingly clear that trans fats were not such a good thing. Regulations were put in place to limit trans fats in food, putting the kibosh on all those foods made using hydrogenated vegetable oils. This is a huge list, including margarine, shortening and anything made with these, which includes countless processed foods: crackers, chips, cookies, pastries and bakery products, sauces, convenience foods, fast foods, and on and on. Peanut butter was frequently mixed with hydrogenated vegetable fat to prevent separation while maintaining spreadability.

Now nutrition labels must list trans fat content. Foods with less than 0.5 grams of trans fat per serving can list "0" as the content, even if there's actually 0.4 grams. Considering that serving size isn't necessarily what you eat, you can consume significant amounts of these fatty acids from various foods throughout the day. If, for example, margarine says 0 grams in 1 teaspoon, but actually contains 0.45 g, and you eat 1 tablespoon on your toast, you've consumed 1.35 grams, which is about 12 calories worth. The recommended limit on trans fats is 1% of your total daily calories. If you eat around 1500 calories/day, that means only 1-2/3rd grams/day. And if food labels don't tell you the whole truth about trans fat content of a food, you could go over that amount, even if you carefully read food labels.

In a world where "0" does not mean *zero*, the easiest way to limit trans fat intake is to avoid foods made with hydrogenated vegetable oils, no matter what the nutrition label says about trans fat content. Hydrogenated oil will be on the ingredients list. At restaurants, fried foods and foods made with shortening or margarine are the most likely to contain trans fats.

As usual, there's a wrinkle in this story. Some foods have naturally-occurring trans fats. Milk is one example, along with anything made with milk, such as cheese. Beef and lamb are also sources. Research suggests that these trans fats are structurally different from hydrogenated vegetable fats, and are not associated with disease risk.

The trans fat saga has resulted in some unintended consequences. Hydrogenated vegetable oils were less prone to oxidation, so the foods made with these resisted oxidation and rancidity. When those foods are made with oils, the foods can spoil more quickly. If you've opened a box of crackers and weeks later noticed an "off" odor, it could mean rancidity, especially if the ingredients list indicates an oil.

Another unintended consequence: the growth of the palm oil industry. Palm oil is naturally more saturated than other vegetable oils, and so resists rancidity and works better in some food products. Foods made with palm oil might be touted as "trans fat free!" or "natural!" (such as in peanut butter). What the labels don't tell you is that giant swaths of tropical rain forest were scraped off to make way for the mono-culture palm plantations.

Trans Fats Summary

1. Trans fats produced by the hydrogenation of vegetable oils are linked to increased risk for heart disease.
2. Small amounts of natural trans fats are found in dairy and red meat, but are not linked to disease risk
3. Food labels list trans fat content, but values less than 0.5 grams can be listed as "0", which can be misleading.
4. It's fairly easy to limit your trans fat intake by avoiding foods made with or cooked in hydrogenated vegetable fats.

Take Away on Fats

Now that you know more than you ever imagined about the biochemistry of fats, what are the important points? Here's one thing I haven't mentioned yet:

Fat makes food taste good!

And when you get right down to it, we eat food that tastes good. One reason no one can stick to a low fat diet for long is that it just doesn't taste good. This explains why people find a higher-fat Mediterranean style diet much easier to follow long term. Not only does fat improve taste, it's satisfying. Fat slows digestion. You don't feel hungry so quickly. Anyone who's partaken of a large high fat meal knows how that feels – think Thanksgiving, loaded with gravy, sauces, mashed potatoes and desserts with whipped cream. But that type of extreme isn't necessary for the satiating effects of fat.

Here are some other important nutrition-focused take-aways on fat in your diet:

1. Most of your fat intake should be from plant foods: olive oil and other vegetable oils, nuts and nut butters, avocado. Yes coconut is a plant, but the fat is highly saturated, although the primary fats are medium chain.

2. If you eat a plant-based diet, you automatically limit intake of animal-derived fats, which are primarily saturated. Red meats, butter, cheese and cream shouldn't be dietary mainstays, but complete avoidance isn't necessary for most people.

3. All fat is high calorie. If you're trying to gain or maintain weight, adding small amounts of fat to foods here and there – for cooking, sauces and salad dressing, or added to casseroles – can boost calories. If you're trying to lose weight, drastic restriction on fat may backfire if it leaves you feeling hungry. Moderate fat with overall portion control is a better plan.

4. The jury is out on many key aspects of fat and nutrition. Is higher fat intake healthful? Are omega-6 PUFAs inflammatory? Are saturated fats all unhealthy, or just some specific ones, or only above certain intake levels? Are shorter chain saturated fatty acids, such as from coconut oil, actually beneficial? Or is that claim just marketing hype?

19 POPULAR FOOD FEARS

Fear of food is rampant in our culture. We fear carbs. We fear salt. We fear food technology. We fear high fructose corn syrup, but strangely think sugar is OK. Research is badly reported in the Main Stream Media, and more hysteria erupts over things that are really quite inconsequential. We can keep adding to our list of food fears, or tune it all out, and end up cynical, ignoring all nutrition or health advice because we expect it will change tomorrow. Neither of these are good outcomes.

Here are some brief summaries of the current state of affairs regarding some of the most popular current food phobias. It's best to have the facts, and you can make your own decision about whether or not to avoid any of these.

GMOs

Genetically Modified Organisms are plants or animals produced using genetic technology, inserting genes into an organism to confer a growth advantage. Genetic engineering is used to make plants more resistant to pests or diseases, reducing the use of pesticides or other agricultural chemicals. GMO plants may also grow more vigorously. A newly approved GMO salmon grows more quickly than other salmon.

All kinds of arguments have been raised against genetic engineering, including the possibility that genetically engineered plants will escape into the wild and alter the gene pool in other plants. Some people think GMOs are actually additives (they are not) or toxins (they are not). Some people just don't like the idea of messing with genes. There is an active anti-GMO movement, demanding that foods be labeled if they contain any trace of an ingredient from a GMO food source.

Let's say some GMO corn is grown, harvested and processed into corn syrup. The resulting corn syrup is used to sweeten a candy bar. In some states, that candy bar must be labeled "contains GMO" or something like that. But what does the candy bar actually contain that's GMO? Nothing. The corn sweetener came from a GMO plant, but is otherwise indistinguishable from corn syrup from other sources. Non-GMO corn syrup is still calories. It's still a sweetener. Not any healthier.

Application of GMO technology in our food supply is still at early stages. Someday a GMO tomato may be engineered that tastes as good as a fresh summer tomato from your backyard garden, loaded nutrients and free of pesticides. Will you avoid it because it was genetically engineered? Some people would say yes just on principle. Other people will choose based on flavor and price.

Respected publications like National Geographic Magazine have published articles that recognize the importance of technology to the future of our food supply. The planet will have to feed billions of people. More sustainable agricultural practices must be combined with better land management, better management of soil and water, and inclusion of gene technology. Dozens of Nobel Laureates wrote a treatise a few years ago criticizing the anti-GMO movement, noting that gene technology has the potential to improve agriculture in developing countries that now suffer through crop failures and famines at alarming rates.

What should you do? If you're opposed to genetic technology, you can find foods labeled "No GMO!!" or something similar. Keep in mind, plenty of the foods in the grocery store never contained GMO ingredients anyway. Labeling one brand of almonds as non-GMO is rather misleading, since no almonds are GMO. Here's a list of foods that may be GMO:

    1. Corn (usually corn grown for industrial purposes)

2. Soybeans (again, much of it grown for industrial purposes and manufacture of certain food additives)
3. Canola
4. Sugar beets (the resulting sugar – sucrose -- would be labeled GMO even though all sucrose is chemically the same)
5. Papaya (in Hawaii, which by the way is delicious)

A new variety of apple, Arctic Apple, a potato called the Innate Potato, and a new salmon, Aquabounty, which is grown in fish farms, are newly approved GMO foods. Which brings up an important fact: GMO foods are evaluated for safety and must be approved by the FDA, USDA and EPA before they can be sold to the public. For example, the Arctic Apple variety would be clearly labeled in the apple display, and in some states it would also be labeled "GMO."

One other important point: organic food by definition cannot be GMO food. So if you're opposed to genetically engineered food, buying organic food is a default way to avoid those products. On the other hand, as with organic food, food crops that are engineered to resist pests would not contain pesticide residues either. You would think that was a good thing, but not for some people. It's a confusing situation.

If you wish to avoid genetically engineered food there are several strategies to use when you choose food products:

1. Look for "non-GMO" on the label, although as noted above, many foods are non-GMO anyway, so you might be misled into buying one product over another.
2. Buy organic food.
3. Avoid processed foods, which are more likely to contain additives or sweeteners derived from GMO corn, soybeans or sugar beets.

Artificial Sweeteners

Most of us remember a time decades ago when artificial sweeteners meant saccharin, which was used in a very limited number of foods for diabetics and dieters. In the 1960's, soft drink manufacturers started using cyclamate. Who can forget Fresca, one of the original cyclamate-sweetened soft drinks. After some bad publicity about cyclamate – rodents consuming a dose equal to 550 cans of Fresca/day had higher risk for bladder cancer – the food industry went on a quest for other safer non-caloric sweeteners. Aspartame came next, and was widely used in soft drinks and certain types of foods.

As more and more artificially sweetened products were made, they became more normal, but they still carried the stigma of artificiality. Many of the new low calorie sweeteners are sourced from plants, and can claim to be "natural", which makes for better marketing. Food manufacturers now have dozens of low calorie sweeteners to choose from. Even though they all confer a sweet taste, there is a wide range of chemical structures, making some more suitable to use in certain types of products.

Are they dangerous?

None of these sweeteners are permitted in food without regulatory approval. In the US, the FDA oversees regulation of food additives. The primary test criteria is cancer. Do rodents get cancer after consuming extremely high doses of these sweeteners? If the risk is deemed unacceptable, the sweetener is not approved.

In my opinion, the narrow focus on cancer is problematic. There are countless other health problems that could be caused by any food additives, including artificial sweeteners. While some may not be dire, they could seriously affect quality of life or risk for other diseases. For example, many people believed aspartame caused headaches, but the FDA doesn't care about headaches. Recently a new wrinkle on the impact of artificial sweeteners has attracted attention from researchers, who are looking at the effect of these chemicals on insulin, blood sugar and gut microbes.

You might be puzzled at the idea that a low- or non-calorie sweetener could impact blood glucose. By definition, these are not sugar-based molecules. They are not digested and absorbed as glucose. The theory goes like this: the sweet taste signals the brain and gut that sugar is coming. Digestion gears up to process the sugar. As you know from the section on carbohydrate digestion, insulin production is ramped up to handle the anticipated rise in blood glucose. Except... it never happens. The brain and gut were fooled by the sweet taste.

Researchers speculate that when this happens over and over again, as when a person consumes artificially sweetened beverages or foods every day, the insulin control system becomes dysfunctional. And they speculate that another unanticipated effect is possible: your digestive system expected glucose that never showed up. So hunger signals are sent out, telling you to eat. You might be trying to cut back on calories by drinking artificial sweetened soda pop, but in fact you end up craving more sweets and eating more calories from other foods. Some studies show that high consumption of artificial sweeteners is linked to weight gain and risk for Type 2 diabetes.

No surprise, food manufacturers vigorously dispute these findings. For example, you could argue that artificial sweetener consumption is linked to higher risk for Type 2 diabetes because people at higher risk use non-caloric sweeteners as part of a weight loss diet. The food industry and even health organizations continue to support use of non-calorie sweeteners as a means to reduce calorie intake for weight loss. Ironically, as use of these sweeteners has increased dramatically over the past several decades, the obesity epidemic has worsened.

Another related area of research interest is the impact of low calorie sweeteners on the gut microbiome. Rodent studies have shown that artificial sweeteners encourage growth of microbes that extract more energy from food and enhance fat storage. Human studies suggest that effect is at work in humans as well, but more definitive studies are needed. But it does make you wonder. With all the low calorie sweeteners in the food supply, why are people getting fatter?

Take Away on Low Calorie/Artificial Sweeteners

Choosing to consume products with these types of sweeteners is a personal decision. My personal decision is to avoid them. But I realize some people may believe low calorie sweet foods help with weight control. Drinking an occasional diet soft drink doesn't seem like a terrible choice, and it cuts some added sugar out of your diet.

On the other hand if you are depend on lots of artificially sweetened foods and beverages every day, thinking they help with weight control, yet you can't seem to lose weight, you might want to think about that. It means you are focused on consuming sweet-tasting foods and drinks everyday. Whether or not the sweeteners have counter-productive metabolic effects, that dependence on sweets means you aren't eating other non-sweet foods that probably have lots more nutritional value. If nothing else, your taste buds end up jaded from all those sweeteners. It's harder to appreciate subtle flavors, let alone more complicated flavors of vegetables or grains that aren't sweet at all.

Food manufacturers are well aware of this. Sweeteners are added to all kinds of foods that have no business being sweet, from salad dressings to bread to spaghetti sauce and soup. Most ready-to-eat breakfast cereals are sweetened, some with astounding amounts of sugar. Some have 1 tablespoon of sugar per serving. Even most health halo brands and organic cereals are loaded with sugar.

So occasional use: not a big deal. Chronic daily use: I'd suggested you need to re-think your food and beverage choices. Whether or not artificial low calorie sweeteners affect glucose metabolism and gut microbes, they are hooking you on sweetness in general and possibly skewing your food choices.

Other additives

Humans have been adding chemicals to foods for thousands of years. Preservatives, colors, texturizers and flavors are common. The FDA lists dozens of additives approved for use in food, including things like vitamins, fish protein concentrate, agar, wax, nitrites, sulfites, rennet, polysorbates and carogeenan. For the most part, these are added to processed foods, but plenty of less processed foods contain additives. Flour is fortified with iron and some vitamins; milk contains added vitamins and sometimes added protein; dried fruit may contain additives to brighten the color; bread is treated with dough conditioners and caramel color to create the illusion of whole wheat.

Years ago, all additives were under a cloud of suspicion, as the natural foods movement inspired by 60's culture spurned anything deemed unnatural. Additives were blamed for what was called "hyperactivity" at the time. Countless research studies tried to find a cause-and-effect relationship with additives, to no avail. The hysteria died down somewhat, especially as organic food became more mainstream.

Additives are still with us. They are still evaluated for safety before they can be used in food. Many food manufacturers now try to minimize use of additives, to avoid an ingredients list that looks like a paragraph from a chemistry textbook. Consumers may not fear additives so much, but they do connect a long list of additives to a food product that's less natural. Authenticity is a popular buzzword, so perhaps a food product pumped up with additives seems fake, less authentic.

But that doesn't mean the product is unsafe. Or even that it doesn't taste good. Twinkies, Cheese Doodles, Pop Tarts and Cap'n Crunch Cereal depend on a variety of additives for their flavor, color, texture and long shelf life, but that doesn't seem to deter people from buying them. The giant Pop Tart display in the average grocery store is a testament to that fact. When General Mills recently reformulated Trix Cereal to eliminate bright artificial colors and use dull natural colors, consumers rebelled en masse. Give us our colors!

Should you be concerned about additives in your food? This is truly a personal decision. Here are some arguments:

1. The more processed a food, the more additives. So avoiding food with lots of additives generally means eating a less processed diet.
2. Some additives affect individuals differently. You may know of some intolerance to a certain additive,

such as MSG, and avoid foods that contain it.

3. Use of additives can mask the lack of quality (actual food) ingredients. Salt and MSG can cover up lack of flavorful meat stock in canned soup. Sugar sweeteners and chocolate extract can mask lack of real chocolate in mass produced cookies. Colors, flavors and salt can fill in for real cheese in cheese-flavored crackers and snacks.

4. Many additives used for food preservation serve a very important purpose. Without them, food would spoil more quickly, leading to more waste, potentially dangerous spoilage and less availability.

5. Many additives are nutrients, used to fortify food. Some food fortification is mandatory, such as the iron and vitamins added to flour. Some is marketing, such as the omega-3 added to bread or eggs, or inulin added to sugary cereal to boost the fiber content.

6. Plenty of what the FDA calls additives are seasonings you use in your own kitchen: salt, sugar, herbs, spices, vanilla extract.

7. While additives are evaluated for safety, they are not evaluated for the potential to cause less serious problems. If you believe some additive or other gives you trouble – digestive upset, headaches, etc – you have the option of avoiding it by reading ingredient lists. If an additive is used in a food, it must be on the list. So if nothing else, you will always have access to information so you can make choices.

8. There is still no definitive evidence that any additives cause behavioral problems in children. Of course, you are free to believe that they do and act accordingly.

Take Away on Additives

I'm not opposed to additives in general. They serve useful purposes, especially for food preservation or nutrition. I am opposed to fakery in food, and additives are frequently used to create textures and flavors that fool the palate, or replace more expensive real food ingredients.

I avoid highly processed foods in general, so I don't feel the need to peruse ingredient lists so much. Fresh broccoli doesn't have an ingredients list. Frozen chopped broccoli in cheese sauce does. Who needs cheese sauce that's probably loaded with cheese fakery? If you're worried about additives, you'll spend a lot less time examining ingredients' lists if you buy fresh whole foods as much as possible.

So my personal preference is to avoided foods with lots of additives, because for me it's a sign of a highly processed food. Despite the Trix fiasco, consumers are increasingly suspicious of long lists of ingredients with chemistry set names. Food manufacturers are responding by using fewer additives in suitable products.

20 YIN AND YANG: CAFFEINE AND ALCOHOL

One perks you up; one mellows you out. It's a fair bet that caffeine and/or alcohol feature in the daily life of many older women. Not to suggest that we're lushes or hyper caffeinated nervous wrecks. But at this time of our lives, many of us look forward to a warming cup of coffee or tea in the morning and perhaps a glass of wine in the evening. We meet with friends or family for coffee or wine. In civilized countries around the globe, these beverages are integral to the fabric of life. In the US, there's always a slightly judgmental attitude, especially about alcoholic beverages. It seems we haven't really moved on from Puritanism and Prohibition.

In recent years, health research on alcohol and caffeine has gone in two different directions:

1. Benefits: both caffeine, caffeine-containing beverages and certain alcoholic beverages are investigated for beneficial effects.
2. Adverse effects: alcohol and caffeine in general are investigated for detrimental health impacts.

Certainly excess of both caffeine and alcohol are bad for health. Too much caffeine is not good for mental functioning. The same can be said for excess alcohol. Chronic alcohol abuse has distinct negative consequences for health, including liver damage and nutritional deficiencies that impact brain function, along with social impacts on family life and work.

Caffeine itself can provide some benefits, such as improved alertness and slight improvements in athletic performance.

Caffeine-containing beverages like coffee and tea contain other bioactive chemicals which are suspected of providing health benefits. Likewise, alcohol-containing beverages like wine and craft beers have other components related to health.

Caffeine and alcohol are distinctly different molecules with distinctly different metabolic fates and different impacts on the body. The only thing they have in common is that they're both consumed primarily in beverages.

Caffeine is a methylxanthine alkaloid; the molecule includes 2 nitrogen-containing rings, carbon and hydrogen. It is found in over 60 types of plants, including coffee beans, tea leaves, guarana, kola nuts, yerba mate and cacao.

Caffeine is a central nervous system stimulant, and effects include:

- increase blood pressure
- increase gastric acid secretion
- increase intestinal contractions
- slightly raise metabolic rate
- increase anxiety and jitteriness
- interfere with sleep
- have a mild diuretic effect

For most people, caffeine consumption leads to a certain level of tolerance, meaning increased production of the enzymes that metabolize caffeine. People who drink little coffee may not metabolize caffeine promptly, and so the stimulant effect of a cup of coffee is more pronounced compared to a person who regularly drinks 2-3 cups.

Is caffeine itself healthy? There's no compelling reason to recommend that everyone consume some amount of caffeine every day. It's not a nutrient. You don't need it the way you need vitamin C. Some of the stimulant effects are helpful to some people. There's also some evidence that it may be helpful for people with Parkinson's Disease and might have a protective effect against Alzheimer's disease. Coffee drinking is linked to lower risk for Type 2 diabetes. However, for all such studies, you have to consider whether it's the coffee or caffeine itself, or the diet and lifestyle associated with coffee drinking that creates the benefit.

There are plenty of myths about the alleged harmful effects of caffeine, most of which are debunked by scientific evidence. For example, caffeine is supposed to cause dehydration thanks to a diuretic effect. Except we drink caffeine in watery beverages, which offsets any dehydrating impact. There is also no compelling evidence that caffeine is linked to heart disease or cancer.

There is as association between caffeine intake and osteoporosis and hip fracture in older women. One possible explanation is that high coffee intake – 5 cups or more per day – might increase calcium excretion, although that increase is small and only detrimental if your calcium intake is poor. Another theory is that older women are more sensitive to disruption of calcium metabolism by caffeine. If you have osteoporosis and are a heavy coffee or tea consumer, you might consider cutting back. But simply decreasing caffeine intake will not make up for poor intake of all the important bone nutrients.

Alcohol

The alcohol consumed in drinks is ethanol, one of a larger class of chemicals referred to as alcohols. Compared to caffeine, ethanol is a very simple molecule: 2 linked carbons surrounded by 6 hydrogen and one oxygen atom.

Humans have been consuming alcohol in foods and beverages for thousands of years. In fact, it's likely early humans and other animals shared an appreciation for fermented overripe fruit that contained alcohol. So alcohol was first consumed by accident. Humans developed a taste for it and devised ways to ferment certain plant foods deliberately. As a result, we now have wine, beer and other alcoholic beverages.

Unlike caffeine, alcohol does have calories, 7 calories per gram, more than carbohydrates or protein, less than fat.

Alcohol is metabolized by a specific enzyme system that transforms ethanol to acetic acid, which is used in energy metabolism. The process requires B-vitamins. Certain B-vitamin deficiencies are common in alcoholics, because they have to metabolize so much alcohol, while also eating nutritionally poor diets.

The harmful effects of excess alcohol are well known. Consequences of short term alcohol binges range from intoxication and vomiting to impaired judgment and unconsciousness, followed by a severe hangover. Chronic overconsumption can have other harmful effects including heart disease, cirrhosis of the liver, pancreatitis, dementia, ulcers, neuropathies, hypertension and some cancers, as well as injuries from violence and accidents.

So are they any benefits to alcohol itself? There's a general (if reluctant) consensus among health experts that "moderate" drinking has some benefit. Moderate drinkers have lower risk for many chronic diseases compared to non-drinkers or heavy drinkers. Most notably, heart disease risk is reduced. But is the benefit from the alcohol itself or from the beverages that contain the alcohol? Or is the benefit from the lifestyle that includes moderate drinking?

And what exactly is *moderate* drinking? Here's a collection of definitions. As you can see, it's all over the map:

- Less one drink per day
- 3-4 drinks per day
- 2 drinks for men; one for women

Even the Mediterranean diet pyramid includes a glass of red wine to represent the inclusion of alcoholic beverages in that food plan. Several years ago I read a long essay by a man who studied cultural norms for alcoholic beverages. He was concerned about binge drinking on college campuses and wondered if this behavior was found in other countries. As part of his work, he surveyed Italian immigrants on the East Coast about diet and alcohol use. On an average day, the typical response from an adult woman went like this:

Lunch: pasta, bread, glass of red wine
Dinner: meat, vegetables, pasta, glass of red wine

Red wine was what you drank with a meal. You didn't binge. You had a meal that included some wine, and you got on with the day. You'd probably find this same pattern among people anywhere in Europe. One thing we don't know is the size of the glass used, and the amount of wine poured.   Our glasses, including wine glasses, have gotten decidedly bigger in the previous 20-30 years. If you're pouring into a large glass, it's easy to just keep pouring far beyond a standard serving sizes: a 12-oz beer, 5 fluid oz glass of wine or 1-1/2 fluid ounce of distilled liquor.

Much of the research on benefits of alcohol have come from research on wine, particularly red wine. In addition to the alcohol, red wine contains many bioactive compounds that have potential benefits. The polyphenol resveratrol is one example.

Resveratrol is found in the skin or red grapes, as well as in peanuts, peanut butter and blueberries. Because red wine is associated with lower risk for heart disease, resveratrol has been the focus of research, much of it done on animals or in the lab. It shows some antioxidant potential in the test tube, but humans metabolize and excrete resveratrol quickly, so the potential for health benefits is not clear.   That hasn't stopped supplement manufacturers from advertising resveratrol pills for anti-inflammatory and anti-aging effects.

Craft beers don't have resveratrol, but they can have significant amounts of B vitamins and even fiber and protein, depending on the brewing process and filtration. Lest you think craft beer would make a great meal, consider this: many of them are high alcohol, so if you drink that 12 oz serving of beer, you could be getting twice (or more) the calories in garden-variety mass produced beer.

Cocktails and shots of liquor or liqueurs don't have much to recommend in terms of nutrients, unless the cocktails are made with significant amounts of fresh juice. Even then, most of the calories may come from the alcohol and sweeteners. And given the trend towards supersizing alcoholic drinks, those calories can be extreme. A couple of drinks at happy hour could set you back 500 or 600 calories.

Most people aren't thinking B vitamins or calories or even resveratrol while enjoying a drink. Alcohol can sooth or put you in a good mood. Those effects can be significantly positive for mental health, as long as you don't overdo it. Key word: "overdo".

For older women, alcohol can be especially problematic. According to an article on the website of the National Institute on Alcohol Abuse, older women are especially at risk for alcohol abuse. Why? One of the main arguments is that women outlive spouses and end up living alone, and ensuing loneliness can lead to excess drinking. Another argument is that older women have reduced capacity to metabolize alcohol and so feel the effects more acutely, even at low intake. A third argument is that medications can impact alcohol metabolism or alcohol can interfere with medications.

The second argument – reduced ability to metabolize alcohol – is a valid concern. The alcohol stays in your system longer. You may have noticed that you just can't drink much anymore without feeling the impact. Hopefully your wise response to that realization was to cut back intake. The interaction of alcohol with medications and diseases is also valid, and is something you need to review with your prescribing physician and/or pharmacist.

There's another very valid concern about alcohol and aging: dehydration. Alcohol is dehydrating, and unlike caffeine, we typically do not consume alcohol as part of a very watery beverage, which compensates for the effect. Given that we're more prone to dehydration as we age anyway, the impact of alcohol is increased. Drinking plenty of water can help, especially including water when you are also consuming alcohol, such as at a meal. But drinking water or other non-alcoholic beverages will not cancel out adverse effects of excessive alcohol.

As for loneliness leading to alcohol abuse, obviously this is an individual reaction, not at all inevitable. There are plenty of unproductive or destructive choices a person can make when dealing with loss or other personal problems. Alcohol may be one of the coping strategies. It may be temporary or it may turn into a permanent problem.

If, after reading this chapter, you're wondering if you are chronically drinking in excess, you should think about finding help. Trusted family members or friends might be a good source of help and support. Your physician or psychotherapist (if you have one) or clergy are appropriate choices, too. Emphasis on the word "trust". This type of problem can be distressing and you don't want to add the stress of working with untrustworthy or judgmental people to the situation.

Take Away on Alcohol:

Good points:

Some known or suspected health benefits with moderate consumption.

Enjoyable and mood enhancing

Bad Points:

Excess intake leads to many adverse health effects

Older women may be especially susceptible to impact of alcohol due to reduced metabolism

Some older women may be more susceptible to developing alcohol abuse problems

Even moderate intake increases calories

What to do?

1. If you enjoy alcoholic beverages, you don't have any pre-existing conditions that preclude alcohol consumption, and you can honestly say your consumption level fits the definition of "moderate", then enjoy!
2. If you don't care for alcoholic beverages, no need to start drinking now.
3. If your consumption level is higher than the moderate definition, you should reconsider that. Especially if it's a daily thing, rather than occasional. It's not just the alcohol that's a concern. The alcohol would be crowding out actual food with nutrients, so

your whole diet ends up unbalanced, while you're overloaded with alcohol.

4. Beware of large sugar-sweetened cocktails, for the empty calorie load if nothing else.

21 SHOULD YOU GIVE UP MEAT?

I've mentioned the health benefits of a plant-based diet so often you might think I'm advocating for a meatless diet. In fact I do not recommend that for older women. Given all the nutritional and health concerns unique to our age group, a meatless diet might not be the best choice, and a strict vegan diet might be a bad choice. I'm probably going to be criticized for that particular conclusion, but I'm sticking to my professional guns, so to speak.

As the author of a book on vegetarian and vegan diets for teenagers, I know what I'm talking about. Vegan diets are devoid of all animal-sourced foods. That means the higher quality protein foods – meat, eggs and dairy -- are off limits, at a time of life when it's especially critical to include adequate high quality protein throughout the day to preserve muscle mass.

Vegans can consume adequate protein if they eat enough total food. High protein plant foods include legumes (particularly soy foods) and nuts. Whole grains have less protein, but do contribute some as part of a mixed vegan diet. Vegetables and fruit are not good sources.

So in order to consume sufficient protein to build and/or maintain muscle mass, an older person would have to eat plenty of beans, soy and nuts all day everyday. Not a problem? Perhaps not for young people who eat plenty of calories and can consume adequate protein by default. When it comes to older women, there's a catch: we need adequate quality protein but fewer overall calories. And plant foods are particularly filling, which could lead to less food intake. It's not a great recipe for protein intake success.

Consider this comparison of foods with equivalent protein:

Food	Protein	Calories	volume
2 large eggs	12.5 g	140	About ½ cup
1.5 oz chicken	12 g	80	1/3 cup
Peanuts	12 g	280	1/3 cup
Kidney beans	12.8 g	190	1 cup

Chicken is the clear favorite, with less volume and fewer calories. Eggs provide the same protein at modest volume and low calories. It's also important to realize that the protein in chicken and eggs is higher quality than that of either kidney beans or peanuts. So you're getting more protein bang for your calorie buck for animal-sourced foods.

There are probably plenty of older women who are vegan who will claim they are perfectly healthy, and I don't know what I'm talking about. If that's you, fine. I'm not going to argue about your choice. I just don't think it's the best plan for older women who need adequate quality protein while eating less food overall.

In addition to protein, B12 is another critical nutrient for older adults. And as noted previously, B12 is only found in animal-sourced foods. Vegans must consume fortified foods or take supplements to get any B12.

If you're opposed to meat, a better choice is a vegetarian diet. This diet is plant-based, but includes eggs and dairy foods, both of which can provide plenty of high quality protein, as well as B12. The added bonus is that dairy foods are high calcium, which is another concern for older women.

Making Vegetarian Work

A balanced vegetarian diet can be a lot like a Mediterranean diet, minus the small portions of meat or fish. Meals are primarily plant foods, with modest amounts of dairy or egg added to boost the protein. The perfect example is beans and cheese. Both of those foods are high protein. The protein in a cup of beans is enhanced by adding a sprinkling of grated cheese, perhaps ¼ cup (about one ounce). The cheese blends in, without noticeably increasing the volume of the dish. You get more protein without feeling stuffed.

This technique works for all meals and snacks. In fact you've probably been eating this way by default at many meals. A breakfast of oatmeal with milk and/or yogurt, dried fruit and chopped nuts is a perfect example. You can probably think of many other examples from the meals you typically eat.

Not all of your vegetarian meals and snacks must contain a dairy or egg food. But if you want to maintain an adequate protein intake, you should be sure some of the foods or ingredients in a meal are good protein sources. Toast with nut butter or a stir fry of vegetables and tofu or a snack foods like edamame (immature soy beans) or hummus are good examples. The option to include eggs or dairy expands your protein choices, as well as the variety of flavors in your diet.

Making Vegan Work

You can make vegan work, but you need to pay particular attention to including high protein plant foods at all meals and snacks, and eating sufficient portions. Remember the 150 pound woman in Chapter 6 who wanted to eat 80 grams of protein a day? What would that look like coming strictly from plant foods? Here's a sample day of high protein plant foods:

1 cup tofu cubes – 18 grams 240 calories
1 cup kidney beans --13 grams   190 calories
¼ cup peanuts – 10 grams 220 calories
½ cup refried beans – 6 grams 100 calories
2 oz dry spaghetti, cooked – 7 grams 200 calories
1/3 cup hummus - 6 grams 140 calories
1 cup cooked brown rice – 5 grams 220 calories
2 cups plain soy milk – 14 grams 220 calories

The protein total is 79 grams at a cost of over 1500 calories. If all you eat is 1500 calories, there's no room left for anything else. No vegetables or fruit or bread, no salad dressing or sauces or sweets or fats used for cooking. Also possibly no room in your stomach for anymore food. So you see the dilemma. Getting significant protein only from plant sources is difficult. For many older women, it will be impossible, because it's hard to eat that much of those types of foods Every Single Day.

You could resort to using protein powders. Soy, pea and other protein powders are available and can be mixed into smoothies. You could buy processed soy burgers, which might be more convenient. The main message: if you want to be vegan, you need to pay special attention to your protein sources every day, while maintaining dietary balance with a variety of foods. There won't be much room in your diet for treats.

Take Away Message

Vegetarian diets are feasible for older women, as long as you include dairy foods or eggs at your meals and snacks throughout the day. Vegan diets, while not impossible, will be trickier to implement to ensure adequate protein.

22 PUTTING IT ALL TOGETHER

It's all about food. It gives us pleasure, satisfies us when we're hungry and is the focus of holidays and social events. Plenty of people enjoy reading cooking magazines and cookbooks and preparing food at home. The food industry is responsible for the employment of millions of people. Food brings people together and can put a smile on your face. And food is our best source of nutrients.

While previous chapters focused on the impact of various nutrients on health and quality of life, that focus does not imply that you should just take a bunch of supplements and call it a day. Food contains many substances besides vitamins and minerals that are important, from antioxidants to fats to fiber. Yes you could find capsules with fruit powder or fiber tablets or containers of whey protein powder, but why not just eat the real food?

This is not a diet book. I do not intend to outline some rigid meal plan for you to follow. I suspect that, like me, at this point in your life you're comfortable with your food preferences and eating schedule. The one thing I do recommend for everyone is a more plant-centric diet. Calling it a Mediterranean style diet is handy, but that doesn't mean you have to switch to unusual foods and start cooking with a bunch of unfamiliar and expensive ingredients. A plant-based diet can fit into most cuisine styles.

Plant-centric basically means less meat, more plant-sourced

foods. It can be as simple as adjusting portion sizes so meat or dairy foods represent less of the volume on your plate. A bigger serving of salad and roasted Brussels sprouts, a smaller piece of chicken. Done. That was easy! Anyone can do that.

My Diet

Inevitably, if I'm out with friends, the assumption is that I only ever order "healthy" foods, whatever that might mean to someone. Far from it! While I generally avoid food that fits my definition of junk, I do not eat a pure healthy diet. That sounds dreary, like too much work.

At home, my go-to list of foods is something like:

Coffee, bread, yogurt, salad. Repeat.

Well, that's not all I eat. There's also cheese, cereal, milk, potatoes, burritos, fresh seasonal fruit, pasta, the occasional hamburger, eggs, tuna, peanut butter, pizza, chicken and chocolate. Olive oil of course. Cookies, wine, ice cream and the occasional piece of bacon. What more does a person need other than maybe birthday cake?

The Boring Balanced Diet

We've heard about the mythical "balanced diet" all our lives. Health experts still use the term, although the definition is so unclear as to be practically meaningless. The visual representation used to be a plate with a large piece of meat, a tiny pile of boiled green vegetables and a bigger pile of potatoes, with a glass of milk alongside. In the era of plant-focused eating, we get advice like "half your plate should be covered with vegetables". But if you don't eat a meal off a plate, then what? And does a pile of iceberg lettuce leaves count?

When it comes to diets, people want rules, boundaries and guidelines: eat this X times a day; never eat that; eat 2 ounces of that at lunch once a week; these foods are 'toxic'; etc. So while dietary balance is an important concept, we need a new way to describe it so the average person can relate. My current preference, for health purposes, is the plant-based or Mediterranean style diet.

Oldways Preservation Trust worked with the Harvard School of Public Health to develop the most widely used Mediterranean diet pyramid. In the updated version (at oldwayspt.org), the foundation of the pyramid includes all plant-sourced foods: vegetables, fruit, nuts, legumes, grain-based foods like bread and pasta and vegetable-sourced oils. That's quite a range of foods. This section takes up 60% of the pyramid shape. Well over half the volume of foods you eat should come from plant sources, whether from fresh salad vegetables or the mango pureed into your smoothie or the tortilla and potatoes in your burrito.

In my opinion, there's a significant problem here: lumping all bread, pasta and grain foods in with vegetables/fruit/nuts/legumes and oils. Technically that means you could avoid all of the latter foods and eat nothing but bread, cereal and pasta and feel like you were eating a plant-based diet. Technically true, but it wouldn't be balanced. It would be very one-sided, missing significant nutrients that are unique to vegetables, fruits, legumes and nuts.

I have another problem: the emphasis on fish/seafood. This section takes up 20% of the pyramid. So approximately 1/5th of your diet should be fish/seafood. Unless you happen to live along the Mediterranean shore, this is a *huge* amount. Given the sorry state of ocean fisheries, with severely depleted fish stocks, it's bordering on irresponsible. Not to mention, fish is extremely expensive, especially in places far from the ocean. So not only potentially irresponsible, but also somewhat elitist.

What to do? You'll find my concept for a pyramid on the next page. The scale is a rough estimate of the importance I'd give to different types of foods. It's still definitely plant-centric, but each type of plant food has it's own emphasis, so you get an idea of where they all fit into your daily or weekly food choices. I de-emphasize fish for the reasons I gave above. Instead I group all the high protein animal foods together. If you love fish, fine. If you follow a vegetarian diet, that group will include only eggs and dairy foods. If you're vegan, that animal food group goes away and the vegetable/legume and grain groups should expand upward to fill in the protein food gaps.

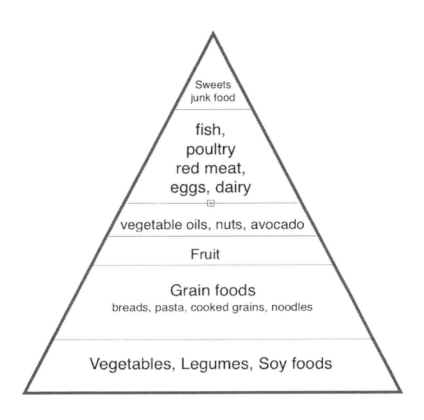

The other reason I wanted to give some emphasis to high protein foods is the need for older women to stick to a consistent intake of quality protein foods to support muscle mass. Despite anti-meat rhetoric, I don't see a problem if you prefer red meat to fish or chicken to eggs. You don't need enormous portions of any of these foods. If meals include high protein plant foods like legumes or nuts, the amount of meat, fish or dairy can be lower, used more as a condiment or for the flavor. Think about the way you might add chicken to a burrito or ground meat to spaghetti sauce. You aren't using 1 lb steaks, you're using small portions, maybe 2 oz per person. That's the kind of meat eating that fits well with a plant-focused diet.

Does this mean never eating a steak or grilled chicken or

fresh-from-the-sea ahi tuna again? No, but it does mean that large portions of meat are not a daily or perhaps not even a weekly thing. If you want to enjoy a large portion of meat or fish sometimes, perhaps it's only once every few weeks. The rest of the time meat and fish are used in small amounts. Meals with large portions of meat can be balanced out with meals that have no meat.

What does this look like in terms of actual meals? Here are some examples:

Breakfast: 2 egg omelet with vegetables, toast.
Lunch: salad with grated cheese/nuts
Snack: cheese slices, whole grain crackers, pear slices
Dinner: burrito with cooked chicken, sautéed potatoes and peppers, salsa, chopped tomatoes, grated cheese

Breakfast: oatmeal with nuts and dried fruit, milk or yogurt
Lunch: turkey sandwich with lettuce, tomato and other fresh vegetable garnishes, fruit salad
Snack: small tortilla with refried beans, grated cheese, salsa
Dinner: pasta with marinara sauce, meat optional, grated cheese, salad

Breakfast: toast or bagel, yogurt, seasonal fresh fruit
Lunch: cheese pizza with vegetables
Snack: hummus dip with celery sticks
Dinner: vegetable soup with beans, added meat optional, bread, salad garnished with pecans

Breakfast: low sugar cereal and milk/yogurt, banana or berries
Lunch: tuna salad, raw vegetable sticks, pita bread or other artisanal bread of muffin
Snack: small yogurt and fruit smoothie
Dinner: stir fried vegetables with tofu, chicken or fish, rice.

These are just some very basic ideas to illustrate the point that eating a plant-based diet is not unusual. Many of us eat that way by default. If you like cooking, you should experiment with recipes to liven up your meals. There are all manner of interesting meatless recipes that use different legumes, seasonings, grains, vegetables and fruit. If you rely on take-out, you can find plenty of similar options, at both specialty grocery stores and restaurants, and, increasingly, at large grocery chains.

If you want rules:

I do have some unofficial food rules for myself. I have an informal list of stuff I would never consider eating. These are foods that don't really contribute much of anything positive to my life or health, so why eat them?

- Snack foods
- Soft drinks, including sports and energy drinks
- Commercial/packaged cookies
- Energy bars
- Commercial/packaged cakes and pastries
- Sugared cereals
- Sugary coffee or tea drinks
- Coffee creamers
- Yogurt that's junked up with additives to create a solid/gelatinous texture, or worse, added candy bits or granola
- Gelatin desserts
- Margarine
- Cured/processed meat products like bologna and similar items
- ***Anything*** artificially sweetened
- Foods engineered to be low fat versions of real food, like low fat cheese, ice cream, salad dressing or whipped topping. I do not refer to foods from which the naturally occurring fat has simply been removed, such as milk or yogurt, or meat bred or trimmed to be lower in fat.

Avoiding this stuff saves money and time. There are now

several entire aisles of the grocery store I don't have to walk down.

I have my own list of super foods. I endeavor to eat these everyday, although I'm not always successful:

- Raw or cooked vegetables
- Fresh seasonal fruit
- Yogurt
- Milk (on cereal) or cheese
- Bread, typically whole grain/artisanal types. In my case, home made 80% of the time because I like to bake
- Water
- Olive oil

I'm less adamant about legumes, nuts/nut butters, eggs, cooked whole grains, meat and fish. In fact I rarely eat fish anymore. I love fish, but the cost, freshness factor and environmental issues are a major concern for me. My preference for meat now centers on sustainably raised varieties. Local is also important whenever possible.

This brings up a nutritional dilemma. High fat fish like salmon, mackerel, and sardines are our best natural sources of omega-3 fatty acids. After reading through the sections on omega-3 fats and health (brain, eyes, inflammation, etc), you understand the critical importance of these unique fatty acids. Where else to get them? The chemical form from plant sources (canola, flax, walnuts) is less biologically effective. My personal/professional choice is to take supplements. As far as I'm concerned, omega-3s are that important to me.

There's a widespread assumption in my profession that supplements are unnecessary, that nutrients should come from food. And that's a nice idea. It's feasible if you eat a lot of food. But in this situation, it's not realistic. The other catch is that, for older women, eating less food overall impacts our intake of all nutrients. We're at the leading edge of a time in human history when people are living much longer lives, and supplements need to be considered a reasonable part of healthy aging. The longer you live, the less you will be able to get all your nutrients from the food you eat.

What's Important?

You might be wondering, after processing so much information about the role of nutrition in healthy aging: what's *really* important? As I wrote the book, I thought about that myself. What I learned about some of the topics made me more conscious about what I eat or don't eat. Here's a short list of the issues I believe have the most potential for a positive impact on your health and quality of life.

Consistent Adequate Protein.

While writing Chapter 6 about protein and sarcopenia, I increasingly realized that this was an extremely important issue that few of us appreciate. And that includes our physicians. There's an unfortunate tendency to just write things off to old age: *Oh well, you aren't as strong as you were 20 years ago, that's life.* Increasing debilitating frailty is seen as the inevitable norm. But it turns out there are metabolic explanations for at least some of the decline in muscle mass and strength. And those metabolic changes can be lessened by consuming more protein throughout the day. Not vast amounts, not necessarily all from animal-sourced food. But consistent.

Frailty is one result of reduced muscle mass. It sets you up for falls and injury, which can have devastating consequences. We'd all rather avoid that. Adequate protein intake helps you maintain muscle mass, and should be part of your strength strategy.

Finally, protein is also critical for other aspects of health, from bone strength to hair and skin.

Exercise

Protein is important for strength, but challenging muscles to work is necessary, too. Muscles don't simply grow in the presence of more protein building blocks; growth must be stimulated by muscle work. And yes, muscles will respond no matter what your age. You might not develop 6-pack abs or huge biceps like a 25 year old, but you can gain strength, which also helps you maintain balance and stability, as well as endurance.

We're lucky to be aging at a time when the importance of exercise is widely recognized, if not widely practiced. Local rec centers, senior centers and private health clubs have classes and facilities that make training and exercise more accessible. If you don't like the gym atmosphere, you can walk, jog, bicycle, hike, dance or participate in sports.

> Wearables – activity trackers – are a great tool. They can remind/nag you to move more or give you a feeling of accomplishment that keeps you motivated. There can be drawbacks: adding up steps can become an obsession for some people; the calorie counts and heart rates aren't always accurate; many don't measure movement other than steps. Obviously they aren't necessary for you to stay active. If you like using one, fine. If not, no worries.

Many people rely on a variety of movement classes as a fun way to get out and move in appropriate ways, supervised by someone who understands the needs and limitations age might bring. Stretching, aerobics, core strength, yoga, cycling and water aerobics are just some examples. I strongly suggest you take advantage of these activities, if you haven't already, as a way to start moving.

Another option is to work with a trainer, especially if you are going to use weight machines. These can be especially intimidating and confusing if you haven't used them before. It's not rocket science, but it helps to have some initial guidance. A trainer can help you develop a plan to progress to more weight on certain machines as your muscles gain strength.

Finally:

- You don't have to be dripping in sweat to get a benefit from exercise. Movement of all varieties is helpful.
- You don't have to wear pricey or fashionable exercise outfits. Comfortable clothes are the best choice. However, if a fun outfit helps to motivate you, then go for it! There's no law that says cool work-out clothes are only for young people.
- You absolutely don't need to swill sports drinks. If you aren't running a marathon or biking in extremely hot weather, water will do just fine.
- Don't be intimidated by the thought that you might not know what you're doing or that other people are judging you about your clothes or your body or how far you can stretch in a yoga class. This is not about competition; it's about you staying fit and active.

Hydration

The importance of water balance is frequently overlooked. All the talk about drinking water can lead to the assumption that everyone is drinking enough. Does your doctor ask about your water intake? Dehydration can sneak up on you, and cause symptoms that can mimic other medical problems. This is especially true during hot weather or if you're consuming alcohol.

Vegetables: antioxidants, carotenes and fiber

I almost can't emphasize this enough. Vegetables and many fruits are rich sources of nutrients as well as chemicals that provide a health benefit but aren't officially recognized as nutrients. Perhaps they should be. Our bodies don't make phytochemicals, yet the evidence mounts in their favor.

All these substances, along with fiber, provide benefits for eyes, skin, digestion, friendly gut microbes, brain function, heart health and immune function. Anti-inflammatory diets all emphasize vegetables.

Happy Gut Microbes

In the not too distant future, we'll know much more about how gut microbes interact with our digestive systems and influence other body systems, from immune function to risk for chronic diseases to cognition and mood. But why wait? You can act now to encourage healthy bacteria by eating a diet rich in natural fibers. In other words, plenty of vegetables, fruit, legumes, whole grains and nuts. Including fermented foods is also a good idea, whether you prefer yogurt or kimchi. Fiber supplements can never substitute for the variety of fiber you get from actual food.

Supplements

Plenty of my colleagues and other medical professionals are going to disagree with me, but I think certain supplemental nutrients can be helpful for older women. Age and menopause impact physical health in ways that practically demand it. The nutrients of most concern, in my opinion, are calcium, B12, omega-3 fatty acids, vitamin D and minerals like zinc and magnesium. I'm not saying that everyone should be taking all of these. I am saying that, after reading Chapter 12, you'll have information to help you assess your own situation. Have you been tested for vitamin D or B12? Do you have osteoporosis? If so, what is your intake of high calcium foods everyday? Do you eat high fat fish at least twice a week?

Taking a multiple, or half a multiple (my preference) will boost intake of nutrients, aside from calcium and omega-3 fats. However, multiples will still be missing all that other good stuff you get from actual food, substances that simply can't all be packed into a daily pill. Your nutrition game plan has to be food first. Supplements, including multiples, do not cancel out a poor diet.

Healthy fats

Low fat is dead. I'm not the first person to assert that, but I'm adding my professional opinion to the discussion. Low fat diets do not work. Not because, on paper, they don't seem to add up, but because in reality no one can follow them. And when it comes to diets, it's all about what happens when the rubber hits the road. You can make up whatever diet you want on paper, and add up calories and protein and claim it will work, but if no one can follow it, it's a failure.

The most pernicious effect of low fat has been the proliferation of low fat foods engineered (usually badly) to sort-of mimic real food. "Low fat" creates a health halo for processed foods like low fat cheese, low fat ice cream, low fat cookies, low fat salad dressing and low fat margarine. Consumers buy this stuff and congratulate themselves on eating a healthy diet. There's evidence that people eat high calorie treats to reward themselves for eating low fat foods.

Low fat diets end up being tasteless and weirdly unsatisfying. Research shows that people can happily stick to diets with more fat content. Fat is satisfying. It helps curb your appetite. You don't feel the need to dish up second helpings or pick at sweets after a meal that has sufficient fat.

The catch is that the type of fat is important. I don't recommend that you load up on bacon, fatty beef or processed meats. A little of those is permissible, but vegetable fats are preferable for health. My recommendation is olive oil as often as possible, particularly the extra virgin variety, because the phenols (which give it color) are thought to provide additional health benefits.

So the take away message here: Eat real cheese, just not huge slabs of it. Put real olive oil on your salads with a splash of vinegar. Ditch the cooking sprays and non-stick pans and use oil for cooking. If you eat meat, worry less about the fat content and more about total portion size, which should be small-to-modest. High fat treats should be occasional and in small portions. Honestly, if you use so much whipped topping that buying low fat versions makes a significant difference in your calorie intake, then you have a bigger problem – your whole diet is 'off'.

Less added sugar and sweeteners

In my opinion, sweeteners have spiraled out of control in our food supply, and I include artificial sweeteners in that category. We're increasingly trained to think that *everything* needs to have a sweet kick built into the flavor mix. Soft drinks and desserts are just the obvious examples. It's practically impossible to find a ready-to-eat cereal that does not have added sugar. Salad dressings have added sugar. Why? Even foods that are supposed to be sweet, such as canned cake frosting or chocolate coated candy bars or cookies now seem to be even more sweet, if that's possible. And along the way, the actual flavor has disappeared.

Certainly high sugar foods like soda pop or cookies add empty sugar calories that you probably don't even need. Avoiding those types of foods as a way to manage your weight is perfectly rational. But (again, my opinion) there's another more insidious effect of adding sweeteners to foods that shouldn't be sweet: we start to expect sweetness. Foods that don't have that little sugar zing start to seem bland. This effect is especially troubling for kids, but it can still affect adults, especially as our taste sensitivity can decrease as we age. We may have less appreciation for a crisp fresh cucumber or a fresh peach, preferring instead salty pretzels or candy.

> **A funny Age vs Taste Anecdote**
>
> An acquaintance was caring for her 80-something mother, preparing wholesome healthy meals. Mom typically picked at the food, eating little. One evening after dinner, the daughter walked in on her mother in the bedroom, munching away on Reese's Peanut Butter Cups. "Why are you eating those?! I cooked you a wonderful meal!" Mom was not amused. "I like these better." The intense flavor of sugary candy was more enticing than chicken, potatoes and vegetables. She wanted the flavor, even knowing it was less healthy.

Enjoying food!

This is what it all really comes down to – eating food you enjoy. Of course, there's a catch. You can think: 'Well I enjoy chocolate and ice cream, so I'll eat those. What could go wrong?' Yes, you should eat food you enjoy, but I'm hoping you enjoy healthy food.

When it comes to flavor, "healthy" food has a bad rap. There's a popular belief that healthy food tastes bad, or is at best, bland. If you believe processed low fat or low sodium or artificially sweetened foods are the norm for 'healthy' then I don't blame you for thinking healthy food lacks flavor, or worse, overwhelms your taste buds with extreme artificial flavors. If your taste buds are accustomed to excessively salty or sweet foods, you'll think foods with less salt and sugar are bland. You won't appreciate a fresh orange compared to the sugary hit of an orange-flavored popsicle. You won't appreciate the rich flavor of homemade chicken stock compared to highly salted canned chicken noodle soup.

Unprocessed foods don't come loaded up with flavor enhancers and other additives. If you're used to a diet of mostly processed foods, you may need to re-train your taste buds to savor the more subtle flavors of whole foods.

Be Proactive!

Nutrition and food are two of your best tools to enhance your health and quality of life. You aren't likely to reverse the aging process or feel like a 25 year old again, but you can make the most of the health you have right now and in the future. I wrote this book for that express purpose: to give women like me information they can use to promote vitality, strength and energy with nutrition.

GENERAL REFERENCES

Dozens of scientific publications were used for the technical discussions in this book. The list would take of several pages and be difficult to read, as most of the web pages have very long complex addresses. While I maintain that list myself, I didn't want to take up more print space with lines and lines of web addresses.

You can find a list of my go-to websites for reliable nutrient and supplement information at the end of Chapter 13. The following are excellent general references for people who want to delve deeper into some of these topics.

CDC Healthy Aging information topics
www.cdc.gov/aging/aginginfo/index.htm

MET scores: Compendium of Physical Activities
https://sites.google.com/site/compendiumofphysicalactivities/home

U.S. Dietary Guidelines 2015
https://health.gov/dietaryguidelines/2015/guidelines/executive-summary/

American Cancer Society
https://www.cancer.org

American Heart Association
http://www.heart.org/HEARTORG/

American Diabetes Association
http://diabetes.org

National Library of Medicine Health Topics
https://medlineplus.gov/healthtopics.html

National Institutes of Health: health information topics
https://www.nih.gov/health-information

National Academies Press: Meeting the Dietary Needs of Older Adults
https://www.nap.edu/read/23496/chapter/2

PLANT BASED DIET RESOURCES

While plant-centric eating isn't all that complicated, a newcomer would probably appreciate some guidance with recipe and meal ideas. Here are some websites and magazines to help you adopt that type of eating style:

www.OliveTomato.com
This website, run by Greek dietitian Elena Paravantes, is dedicated to the Greek version of a Mediterranean style diet. You'll find recipes, food information and other resources.

OldwaysPT.org
Oldways Preservation Trust is an organization focused on promoting traditional cuisines, with a special emphasis on plant-based eating.

FoodAndNutrition.org
Food and Nutrition magazine is published by the Academy of Nutrition and Dietetics. Consumers will find plenty of plant-centric recipes in each issue, as well as discussions of specific foods and nutrition and health topic updates.

www.MeatlessMonday.com
The Meatless Monday website is intended to help consumers ease into a more plant-centric diet by setting aside one day a week to enjoy a meatless dinner. You'll find recipes and menus, as well as general information about plant-based eating.

VegetarianNutrition.net
Vegetarian Nutrition Dietetic Practice Group maintains a consumer-oriented website with information about meatless diets, as well as recipes, menus and nutrition and diet information.

www.MediterraneanLiving.com
The Mediterranean Living website has a wide variety of recipes.

Many conventional food magazines, such as Cooks Illustrated, Bon Apétit and Fine Cooking, now feature vegetarian and vegan recipes and menus.

INDEX

ABOUT THE AUTHOR

Donna P Feldman, MS RDN, has been a registered dietitian nutritionist for almost 40 years, and holds a Master of Science degree in nutrition and communications from Cornell University. She is the author of "Feed Your Vegetarian Teen", and has an extensive background in plant-based diets. She lives in Colorado and writes about food and nutrition on her blog RadioNutrition.com. Follow her food, nutrition and health updates at:

www.FoodWisdomForWomen.com

Facebook @FoodWisdomForWomen
Twitter @DonnaFeldmanRD

Made in the USA
San Bernardino, CA
13 March 2018